# How to Transform Yourself into Any Animal

## A DIY Guide to Surgical Procedures

by
Orca Man

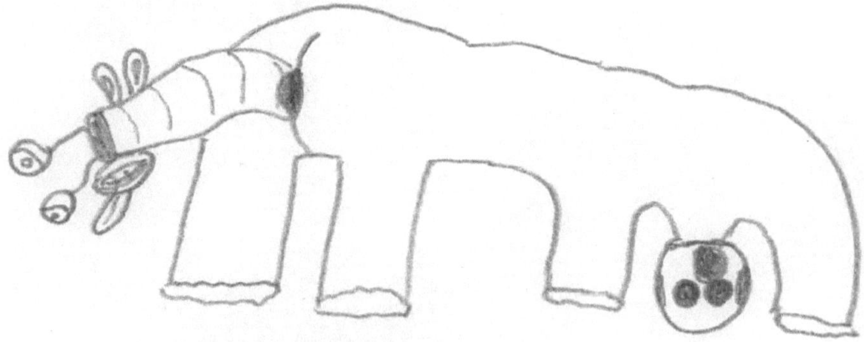

ISBN-13:
978-1507876329

ISBN-10:
1507876327

First print September 2014
Second Edition February 2015

This book has not proof read.

# DEDICATIONS

For John, the best damn blue jay a guy could ask for,

and

Dianne, the only woman I've ever stuffed.

I would like to thank my five year old son Steven for providing the wonderful illustrations for daddy's book. I look forward to Transforming you soon, son.

Glem Jobes, Ben Marinara and Sir Thomas of the James were in no way helpful to me during the course of my writings and should feel deeply ashamed.

This book is specially dedicated to the cast of Saved by the Bell, whose pioneering acting skills blazed the trail for television greatness.

# About the Author

Orca Man's age is irrelevant. The Orca is as timeless as the sea. What is important is that he first Transformed himself in 1991. Since then he has helped others transition from their feeble human forms to glorious new entities. After a court case left him financially challenged and legally unable to physically help others in their transition he was forced to write this book.
He spends his days splashing around happily in his bath tub filled with brine where he hopes one day to raise a family. Whose family that will be he does not yet know.
He has always wanted to get the word "cunt" published.

Important: I, the author lack a fair amount of basic knowledge in human and animal biology. If you spot a mistake or issue in this book then you are most likely correct. Sorry.

I have not included a table of contents as I could not be bothered.

# Introduction

So you've decided to transform yourself into an animal huh? Well congratulations, you've bought the perfect book for you. Unless you stole this book in which case you are scum. Seriously, you make me sick. How dare you? Do you know how long it took me to write this book? You are the worst kind of human being. Now fuck off.

But if you bought this book then please stay. Within these pages lie the surgical secrets you need to completely and permanently modify your human form. To transform yourself into a new entity using practically nothing more than a sewing kit and a hacksaw.

The animal transformation tutorials in this book are split into seven categories:

- Land Mammals
- Birds
- Reptiles
- Amphibians
- Marine Animals
- Invertebrates
- Sea Invertebrates

This will allow you to navigate quickly to the animal of your choosing if you already have your heart set on the one you wish to become. However if you are new to the world of animal transformation and have not decided which animal to become you are advised to read the entire book.
That way you will get a broad knowledge of the severity of each surgical procedure. Everyone has their own tastes and limits when it comes to pain endurance. Remember that in performing these procedures you will be removing part of your humanity and replacing it physically and mentally with a new species. This experience can seem alien and nightmarish to some.
But if you weren't ready you wouldn't have bought this book in the first place. So let's begin.

## Self-surgery vs. Having a surgical partner

It is likely that would prefer to perform your transformation in private and alone. And though it is possible to perform all procedures in this book by yourself the end result may come out sloppy if you are not limber enough.
Therefore it is recommended to have a partner present to help you if know you won't be able to perform tasks like stapling matter to your back or sawing off your own limbs by yourself.
Another factor to consider is pain. Some can work through the pain of self-surgery while others will feel unable to continue operating after pulling out one measly tooth.

If you are that sort of person you should really think about procuring a helper, if only to have someone to hold you down when the screaming starts.

## Anesthetic

Pain killers are NOT recommended when performing your transformation. This may be a turn-off for some but it is for good reason. While anaesthetized you will not be coherent enough to perform the task at hand to the best of your ability. Self Transformation is an art form. You must be lucid and take the pain during your self-surgery. Trust me, you will not regret it when you see the results.
Alcohol is a no-no. You do NOT want to perform surgery on yourself drunk. You'll end up sewing your anus to your shin and that's not good for anybody. Waking up would be the worst morning after of your life.

## Antiseptic

The concept of germs is all witch doctor superstition. The pharmaceutical companies want you to spend your hard earned monies on useless items like bleach and soup. All you need to do is wipe your tools or wound with a damp cloth. It's not rocket science.

# Fighting Blood Loss

Inevitably your Transformation is going to include a bit of spurtage from what is known in the medical community as your blood tubes. Cauterization is the key. Use a soldering iron or regular clothes iron to burn your open, bleeding flesh. Do this regularly – do not ignore a bleeding stump. I know you'll be excited to get on with the next part of your procedure but you won't be able to enjoy it if you die from blood loss.

If you start to feel faint remember **ANIMAL**:

**A**llow yourself to drift into unconsciousness

**N**ote your heart beat rhythm in your head

**I**ndicate you are in trouble by flailing

**M**oan the alphabet to alert passersby

**A**nally discharge yourself as both a sign for help and a treat

**L**ie back and list your life's regrets

# Tools

It is absolutely unnecessary to spend a fortune on sterile professional medical instruments. All tools needed can be found at home or bought cheaply from a hardware store. Another money saving trick is to borrow equipment from a friend. Your buddy Al won't know you're using his power sander to remove your genitals, and what Dave doesn't know won't hurt him.

Here are a few tools you might need:

- Pliers
- Clothes iron
- Soldering iron
- A selection of knives including scalpel and kitchen knife
- Sewing kit
- Super glue
- A bathtub
- A working car or a friend with a working car or a neighbour with a working car who is far too trusting
- Crow bar
- Tar
- Paint
- Staple gun
- A vice
- Power saw
- Power sander
- Sand paper

- Blender
- Scissors
- Plunger
- Syringe
- Bowls of pudding
- Hammer
- Garden shears
- Bicycle pump
- Cheese grater
- An oven. Preferably fan assisted.

## Can't find your animal in the book?

I know the title of the book is How To Transform Yourself Into *Any* Animal but obviously with all the different species in the world it would be impossible to write a surgical procedure for each one.
Luckily this book still lives up to it's name by giving you enough self-surgery knowledge to Transform yourself into even the most exotic entity. Can't find the exact animal listed? No problem. Just find the closest approximation in the book and modify the surgical procedure to your own preferences. A little bit of improvisation and creativity is encouraged and thanks to this book you can fulfil this beautiful dream. So there's no need to ask for a refund, smartarse. Like you'd actually ask for a refund. Go on, I DARE you to fucking ask for your money back. See where that gets you. They would laugh in your face and spit on your back. Which you'd deserve quite frankly. Prick.

# Maintaining a relationship after your procedure

The sad truth is not that many people wanna fuck a porcupine. If you are in a relationship make sure you consult your partner *before* Transforming yourself into an animal. Many of the procedures in this book involve *partial* or *total* loss of *genitals*. That can be a real *deal* breaker for some people.
Getting your partner to *accept* the new animal that you are is the first step to *maintaining your* relationship. The other is planning *activities* for you two to do. Your new physique will *allow* you to do things you and your partner *never* thought *possible*. Being a giant spider opens up a whole new *world* of possibilities in and out of the bedroom. *There are so many new games to play*. On the other hand there are some *things* you just won't be able to do anymore. If you *want to be* a piece of coral your partner will have to accept the fact that both your *lives* will be *limited* to the things coral can *do*.

Authors note: I added a bunch of italics in that section to make it more fun.

# Will performing the procedures in this book kill you?

Possibly, yes.

# Is the author legally liable for this?

No.

# Section 1: Land Mammals

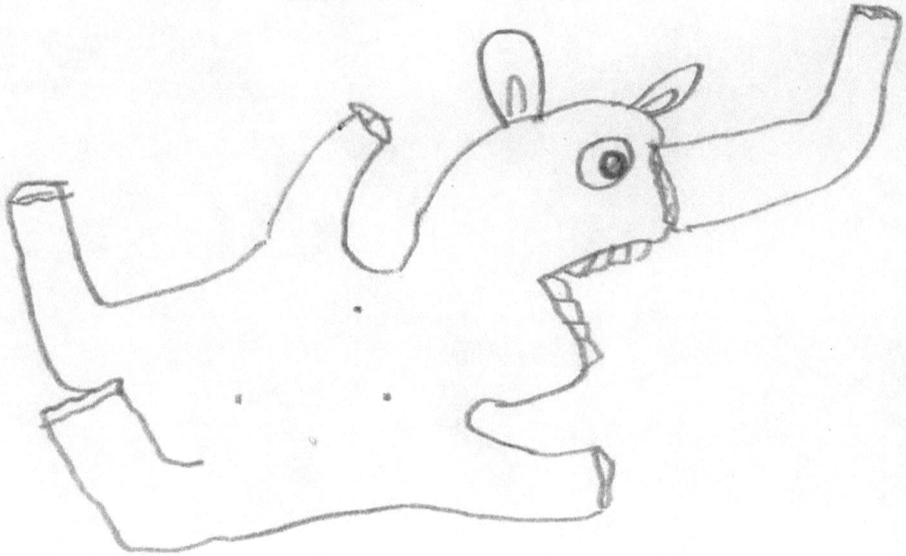

Many land mammals are covered in fur. To replicate this acquire a sack of hair from your local barbers. Pour this and an entire tube of super glue into a bath tub. Then dive in. It is recommended you do this AFTER your procedure. Then use dyes and spray paints to create your animal's markings.

## Aardvark

1. Gently remove spine. This will give you the hunched over look of an aardvark.
2. Stick spine to the bottom of your torso. This is your new tail.
3. Remove scrotum, stretch it out and cut into two long pieces. [If female acquire scrotum]
4. Staple the two pieces of scrotum to your ears.
5. Use tongs to pull out your rectum. Staple this to your nose.

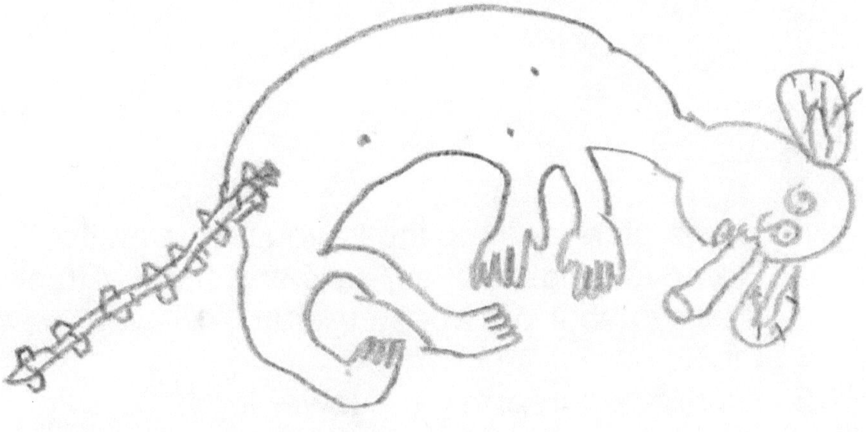

## Armadillo

1. Replicate step 1 and 2 of the Aardvark procedure.
2. Remove all the skin from your body. Patch it into one piece and run a hot iron over it. Leave it out in the sun for 48 hours. Then use a scalpel to score a grid patter all over it.
3. Use hot glue to fuse the skin to your back.
4. Remove entire lower jaw.

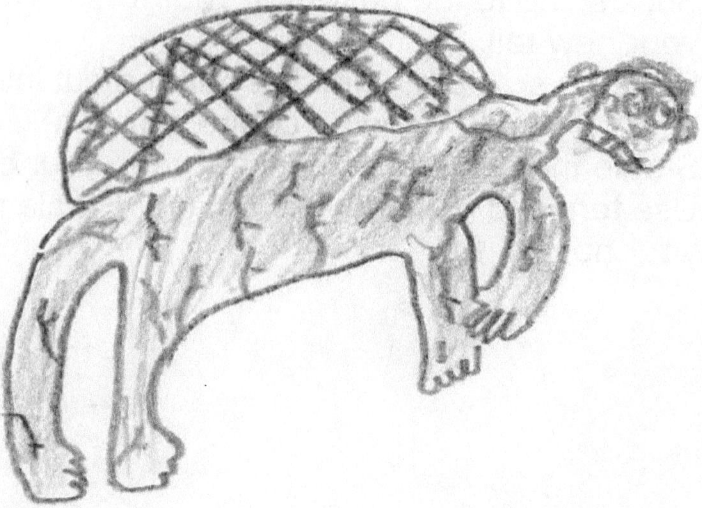

## Anteater

1. Use a plunger to collapse your anus on itself.
2. Remove tongue, eyes, ears and teeth. Attach these to your prolapsed rectum AKA your new face.
3. Amputate forearms and lower legs.

[If blindness does not appeal to you stretch your optic nerve and gently push your still attached eyeballs down your throat, guiding it through your body till it exits through your rectum.]

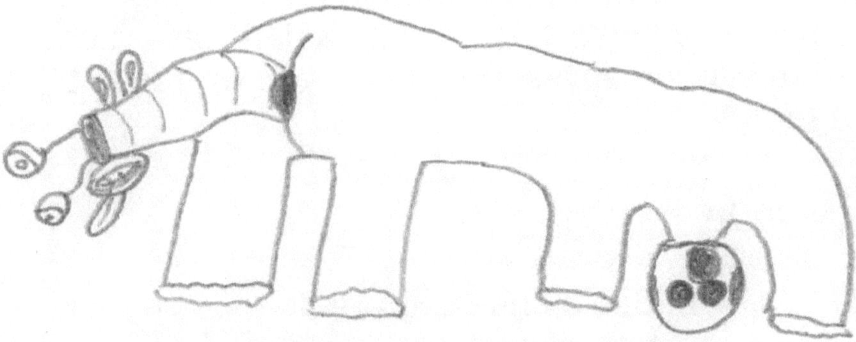

## Antelope

Stick your head in a vice and use it to make your face longer and less wide. Your eyes will bulge, adding to the look.

1. Stretch ears out with pliers.
2. Remove two ribs and hammer them into your skull.
3. Get on all fours.

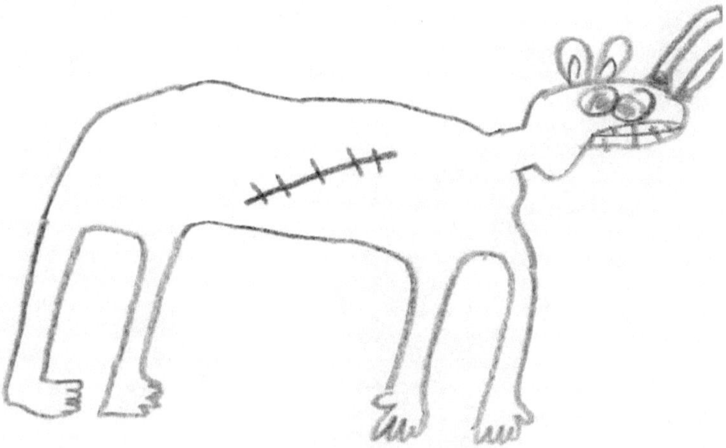

## Aye-aye

I don't know why you'd want to look like this. The best advice I can give you is to find a dark cavern and stare into the abyss. Eventually you will resemble an Aye-aye.

## Baboon

1. Use a cheese grater to redden your buttocks.
2. Remove spine and staple it to the bottom of your torso.
3. Scalp yourself. Cut the scalp into two pieces. Glue these pieces to the sides of your head.
4. Use a vice to elongate face.

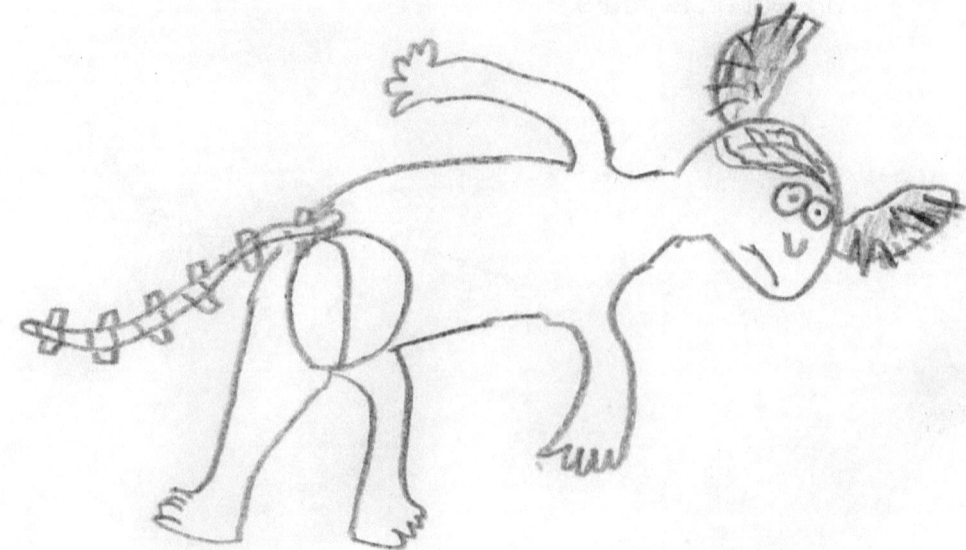

# Bat

1. Replicate steps 3 and 4 of the Aardvark procedure.
2. Remove all the skin from your body. Patch the skin pieces together. Cut this into the shape of bats wings.
3. Remove several leg and arm bones. The specific ones don't matter. Stick these to the bat wing shaped skin to make it look authentic.
4. Use hot glue to fuse the wings to your back and forearms.
5. Dive into a bath tub filled with hot tar.

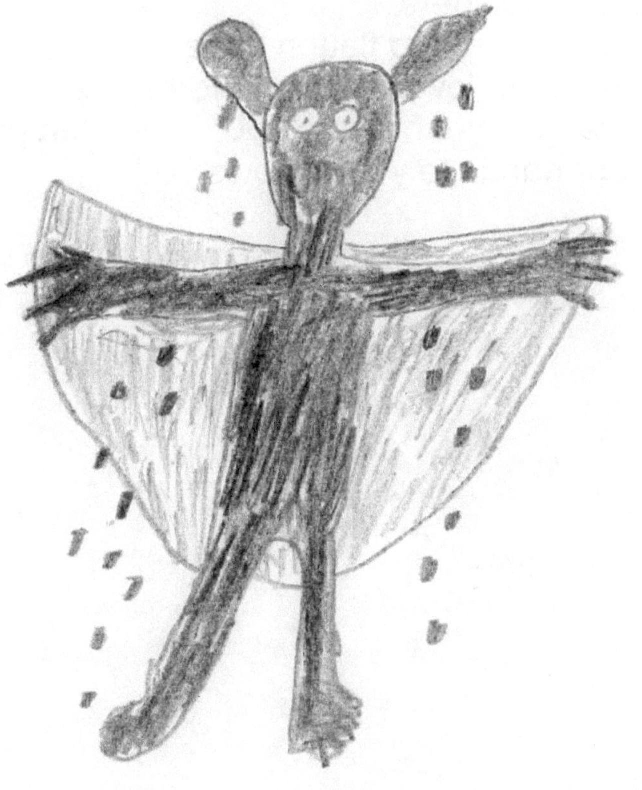

## Beaver

1. Amputate lower legs. Put these in a blender and shape the mashed up flesh and bone into a beaver tail shape.
   Bake for 50 mins at 140 °C / 45 mins if fan.
2. When the tail returns to room temperature staple it to your anus.
3. Use pliers to remove all your teeth. Jam your two front teeth back into the gums before the wounds heal.
4. Very delicately remove neck without decapitating yourself. Then staple your head to your shoulders.
5. Use hammer to flatten nose.
6. Amputate lower legs and forearms.
7. Reattach your feet to your knee stumps and your hands to your elbows.

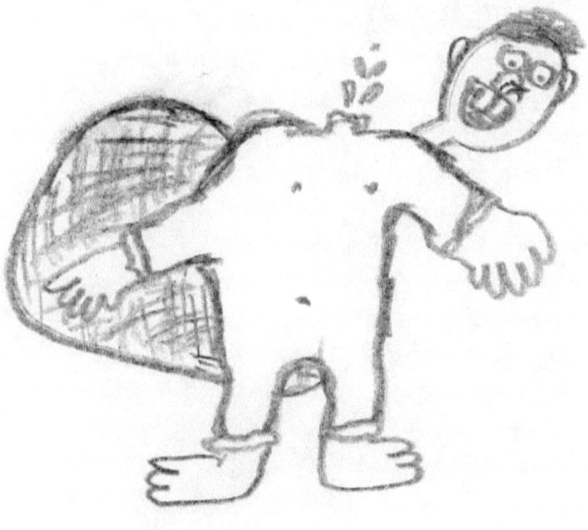

## Bear

1. Use scissors to snip off the end of your nose.
2. Cut off ears and glue them back on to the top of your head.
3. Replicate Step 4 of the Beaver procedure.
4. Cut your fingers off at the knuckle joint.
5. Get a syringe and two bowls of chocolate pudding.
6. Inject your cheeks with the pudding so your face swells, giving you a bear-like look.
7. Grab both of your jaws at the same time and pull HARD. Do this till you break the jaw bone. Now keep pulling to elongate your face.
8. Get on all fours.

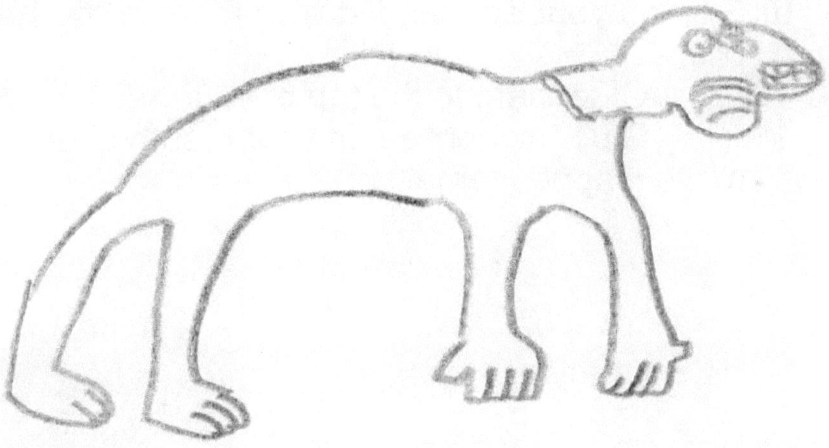

## Bobcat

(See Cat. Add tiger markings.)

# Cat

1. Replicate instructions 1 and 2 of the Aardvark procedure.
2. Cut off all your fingers and toes.
3. Slice off your nose.
4. Remove eyelids and use a bicycle pump to pump air into your eyeballs.
5. Use a soldering iron to change your pupil from a circle to a slit.
6. Remove the flesh from your amputated fingers and toes.
7. Use a sharp knife to sharpen and thin out the bones of these.
8. Now jam them into your face. These are your whiskers.
9. Snip off your ears and stretch them out with pliers.
10. Glue them to the top of your head.
11. Glue the corners of your mouth shut to make it appear smaller

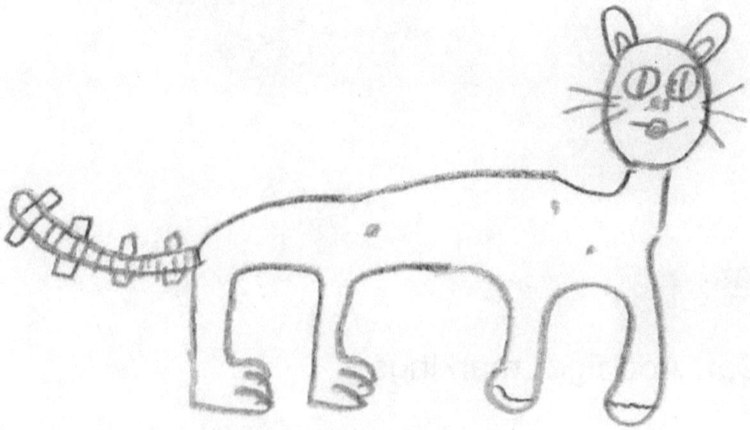

## Cheetah

(See cat. Take speed.)

## Chimpanzee

1. Cut off nose.
2. Draw a circle on your mouth reminiscent of Homer Simpson.
3. Now use a scalpel to score around this circle and peel the skin off.
4. Burn the rest of your face with an iron.
5. Amputate your arms and your legs.
6. Now sew them back on, placing your arms where your legs should be and your legs where your arms should be.
7. Use pliers to stretch out ears. Do not do this if you already have big ears.
8. Slouch.

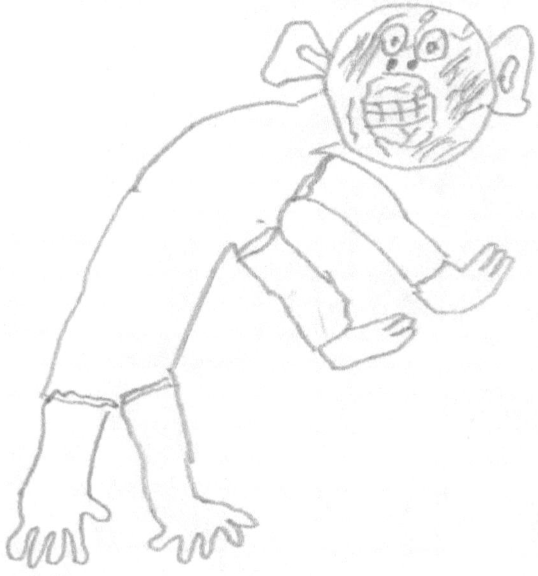

# Chipmunk

1. Amputate legs.
2. Cut the feet off the amputated legs and save them for later.
3. Cut your arms off. Then cut off the hands and staple them to the bottom your body.
4. Now staple your feet to your chest so that they cover up your nipples.
5. Grab one of your amputated footless legs and staple it to the bottom of your back, just above the anus. Cover in fur. (The leg, not your anus.)
6. Completely cut out your bottom jaw.
7. Conceal your open mouth by cutting out a sheet of skin from your other leg. Stitch this to your face so it covers the hole where your bottom jaw used to be.
8. Use scissors to snip off your nose.
9. Snip off ears and glue them to the top of your head.
10. Completely remove spine. You will now have the posture of a chipmunk.
11. Grab two bricks of equal weight and smack them into the sides of face so that they slightly cave in.

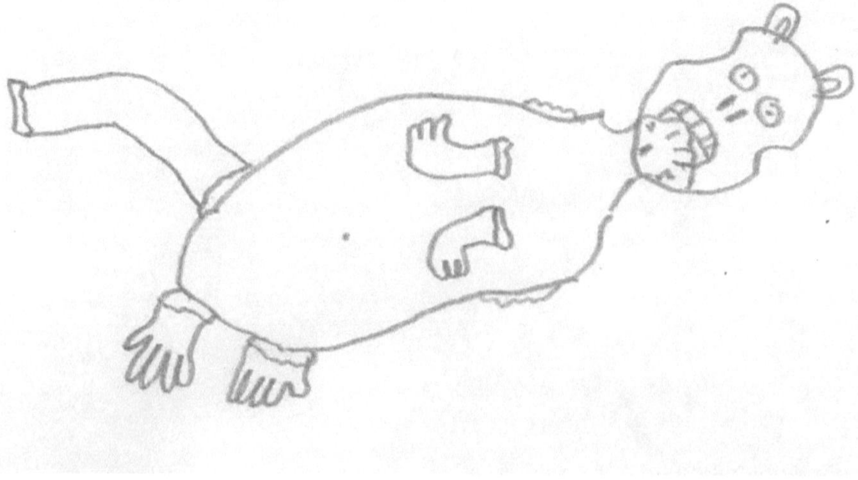

## Cougar

(See Cat. Become muscle bound and dickish.)

## Coyote

Replicate Wolf procedure. Starve yourself.

## Dingo

It's basically a fucking dog.

## Dog

There are many different breeds of dog. Use this procedure to attain the basic shape of a dog and then modify it to your tastes. For instance if you want to be a pug simply whack your face repeatedly with a shovel after the procedure.

1. Cut off your toes, thumbs and fingers at the second knuckle.
2. Snip off ears with scissors, use pliers to stretch them then glue them to the top of your head.
3. Got on all fours
4. Remove a portion of your spine. How much depends on how long you want your tail to be.
5. Glue faux fur to the tail them insert it into your anus.
6. Snip off the pointy part of your nose.

7. Use a hammer to break your upper and lower jaw.
8. Pull the jaws out as far as you can then snap them back into place.

If you want multiple nipples simply glue peperoni slices to your chest and stomach.

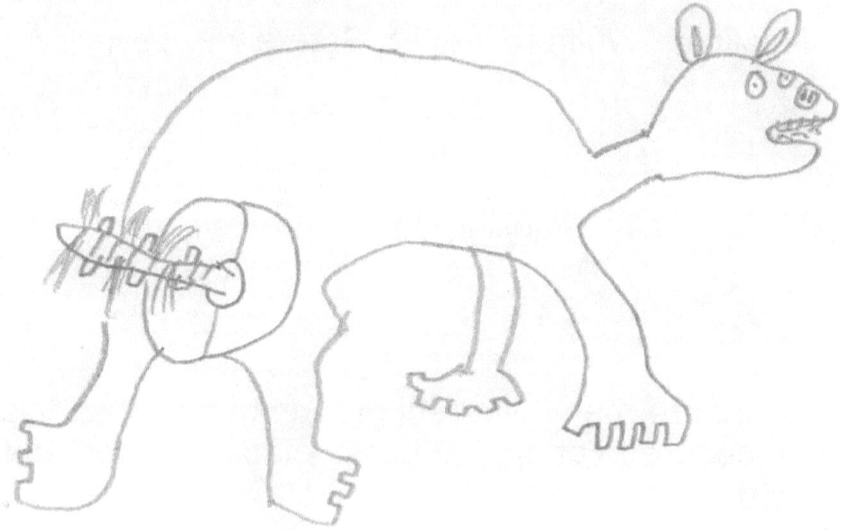

## Elephant

1. Follow the procedure in the Reptile Section on Skin.
2. Completely amputate one of your legs at the hip.
3. Staple this to your face.
4. Slice the skin off your back and cut it into two triangular sheets. Staple these to the sides of your head.
5. Amputate your other leg at the knee.

6. Use this to replace the other amputated leg. Sew it into place.
7. If you want tusks remove two ribs and hammer them into your face.

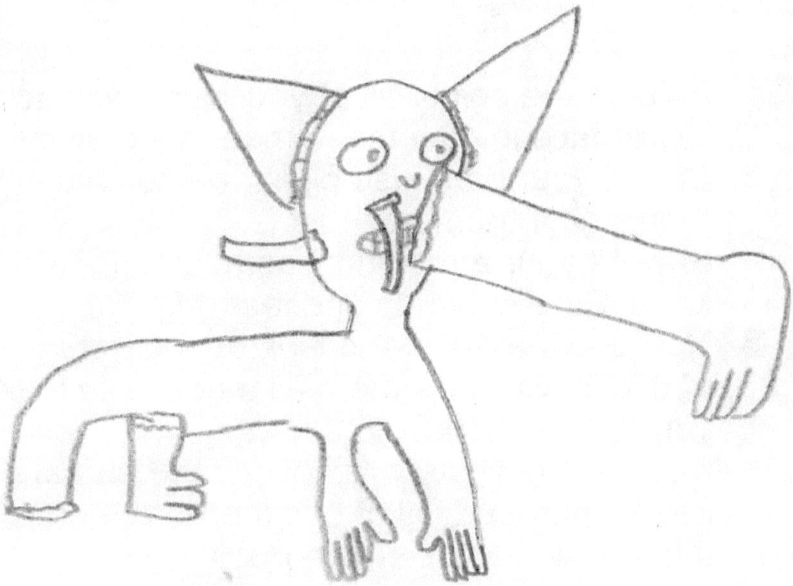

## Elk

(See Moose)

## Fossa

Follow Cat procedure. Spend a week in a dumpster.

## Fox

Follow Dog procedure. Use scalp to decorate tail. Starve self.

## Gibbon

(see Monkey)

## Giraffe

1. Snip off the pointy bit of your nose with scissors
2. Cover face in glue then smear sand all over it.
3. Cut off your ears, use pliers to stretch them then staple them back on.
4. Saw off your arms and legs at the elbow and knee. Cut the hands and feet off.
5. Now line the arms and legs up together in order of thickness. Stick them all together to make your giraffe neck.
6. Now very delicately remove your head and keep it pumped full of blood and oxygen. To do this follow these instructions:
    - Get a bucket filled with the blood of your type.
    - Attach a fish tank filter to the blood bucket.
    - Plop your severed head into the bucket. If it does not float duct tape pool armbands to the sides of it.
7. Sew the giraffe neck to your open neck hole.
8. Get a long bit of rope and tie one end to your severed head.
9. Throw the head up and try to make it land in your neck hole. Think of this is as a man-sized fleshy version of paddle ball. Remember if you don't get the head on in two minutes you risk brain death so time yourself and when needed dunk the head back in the blood bucket.

10. When you have gotten enough practice and are confident you can get the head onto the top of the neck, smear super glue to open neck hole of the head.

11. Throw the head onto the top of giraffe neck and wait for the glue to set.

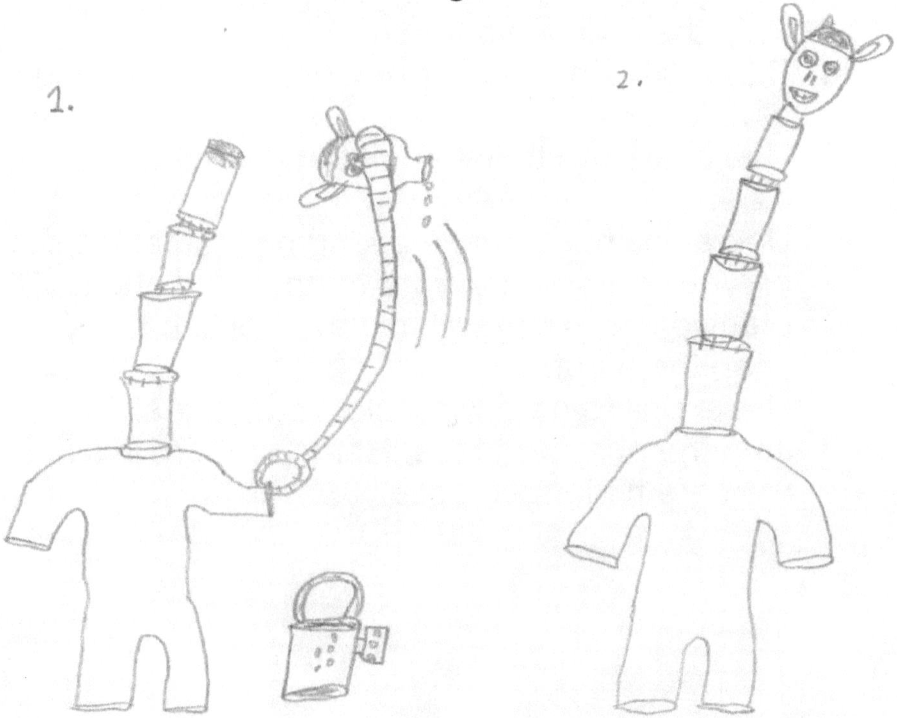

## Goat

1. Amputate your arms and legs at the knee and elbow.
2. Bite on the end of a heavy table and pull as hard as you can till your jaw stretches.
3. Snip the end off your nose.
4. Either grow a beard or procure pubic hair and glue to face.
5. Use a hot iron to flatten out and stretch your ears.
6. Use a scalpel to make a long horizontal incision on your chest. Stick your hand inside and pull out two ribs. They will be firm. You'll have to snap them out.
7. Use a drill to bore two holes into your skull.
8. Jam the ribs into these. Hammer them in till they are no longer loose.

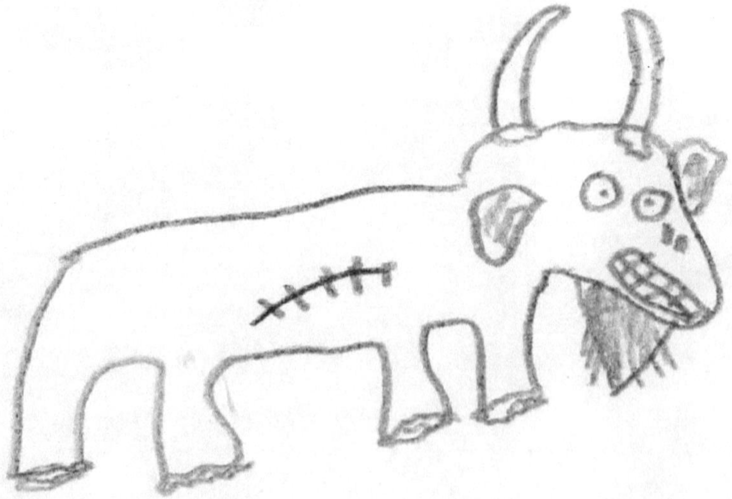

## Gorilla

1. Beg, steal and borrow as much hair you can get your hands on. You need enough to fill a bathtub. The easiest way to get is scrounge the bins at hairdressers. Since you'll need so much it's best to go from town to town, targeting multiple barbers a week. Never scrounge from the same place twice.
2. Coat your entire body in at least five layers of super glue.
3. Dive into the bath of hair.
4. Use scissors to snip off your nose.
5. To give your body that bulked up feeling distress a bee hive and let them sting you all over. Swelling is nature's steroids.
6. Cut off your arms and legs.
7. Now staple your arms where your legs used to be and vice versa.

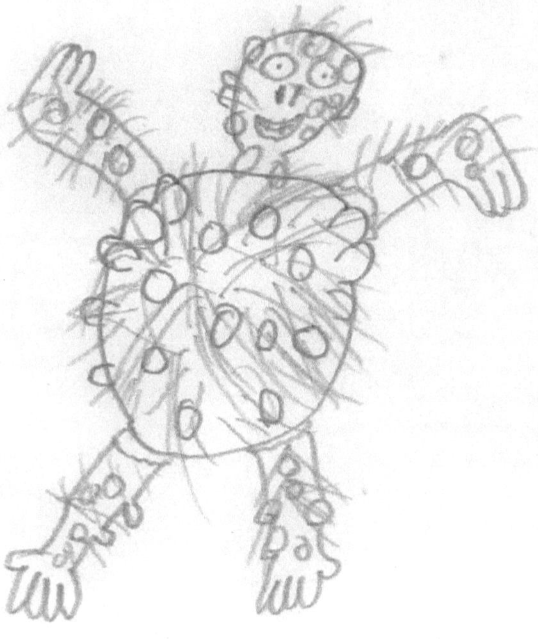

## Groundhog

1. Slice your body in half at the waist.
2. Cut off your legs and glue them to the bottom of your torso.
3. Cut off your arms. Slice the hands off the severed arms and then glue them to your arms stumps.
4. Smack your head against a wall till it appears as if you have no neck.
5. Cut off ears.
6. Nail your bottom jaw to a heavy table. Now pull back hard until the jaw is torn off.
7. Remove all but your two front teeth.
8. Snip off nose.
9. Cut up half a forearm and staple to anus.
10. Glue two dozen fine pubic hairs to your face to give yourself a whisker-like look.
11. Slurp pudding till you get a bit chubby.

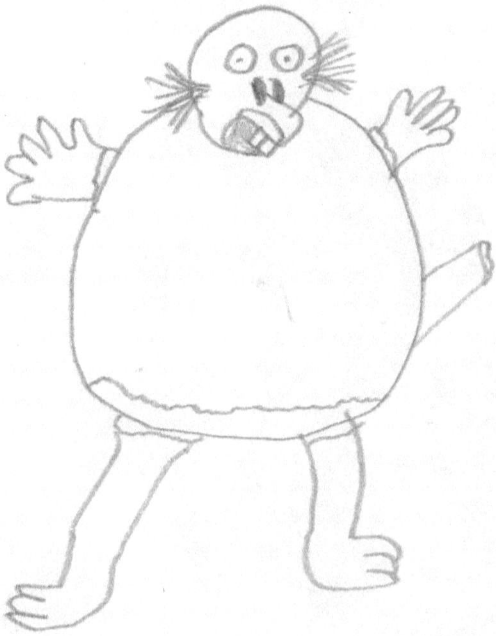

# Hare

If you can honestly tell me the difference between a hare and a rabbit I don't wanna know you.

## Hedgehog

1. Stick your head in a vacuum till it tapers like a round pyramid.
2. Cut off arms and legs at the knee and elbow.
3. Cut off hands and feet and stick back onto the body.
4. Dissolve the arms and legs in acid till they are nothing but bone.
5. But the bones in bleach overnight.
6. Finally use butter to polish the bones.
7. Now get a sledge hammer and smash the bone up into little bits. This would be a fun time to shout "Where is your God now?!"
8. Collect two hundred of the longest and sharpest bone fragments.
9. Stab them all over your body. No need to hammer them in. If they fall out simply re-stab.

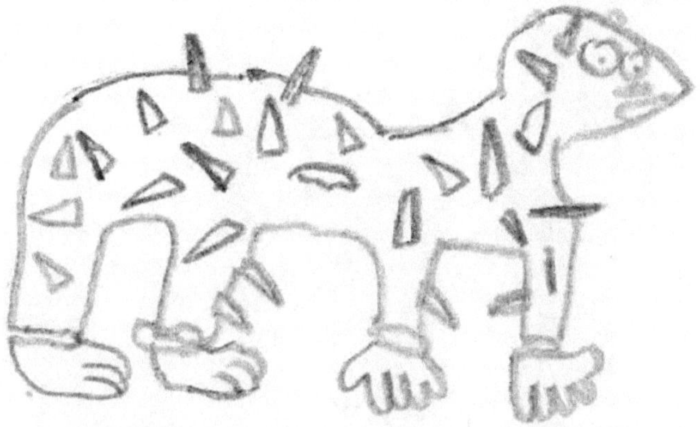

## Hippopotamus

1. Spend a year overeating till you become what can best be described as a fat fuck.
2. Shave all the hair and skin off your body.
3. Lie out in the sun and wait for the exposed flesh to harden and dry out.
4. Use a crowbar to remove your shoulder blades.
5. Sharpen the thinnest end of the blades into points.
6. Stab the blades into your upper and lower jaw. You now have a set of flapping hippo jaws.
7. Cut off ears.
8. Amputate your arms and legs at the knee and elbow.

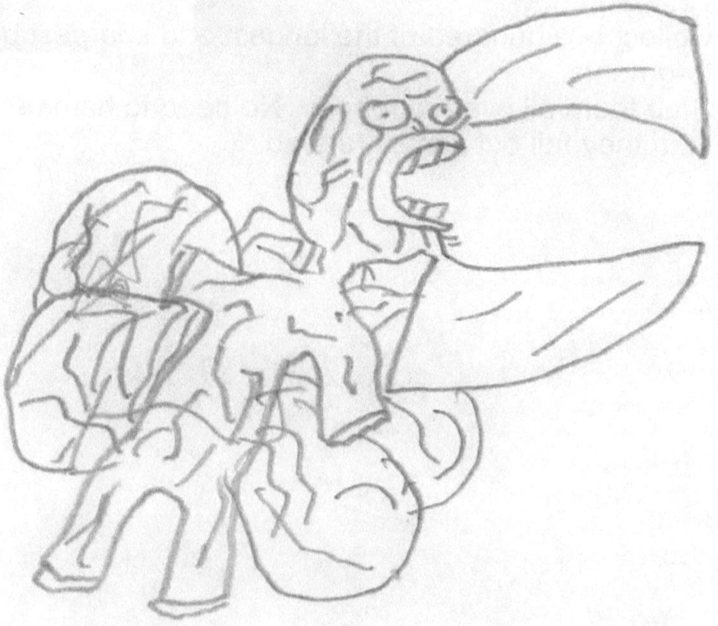

## Horse

1. Cut off your feet. Nail horse shoes into them.
2. Do the same to your hands.
3. Use a vice to elongate your face.
4. Super glue a long bunch of hair to the bottom of your back.
5. Snip your ears off with scissors and glue them to the top of your head.
6. If you want a mane of hair then do nothing. If you don't want a mane then scalp yourself.

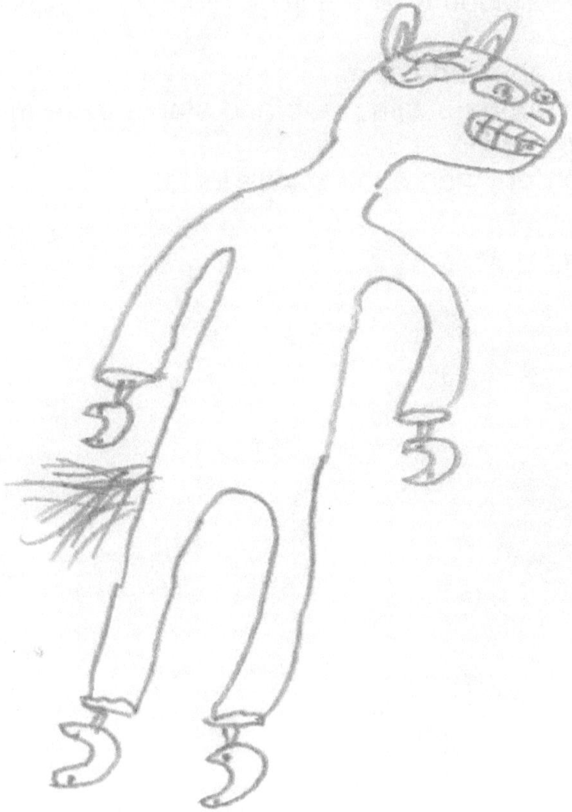

## Jaguar

AKA a LEOPARD!

## Kangaroo

1. Amputate arms and legs. Cut them in half at the elbow and knee. Remove skin and flesh from the lower legs and forearms.
2. Sew lower legs and forearms back onto body.
3. Sew one upper arm and upper leg together. Staple this to the bottom of your back. It should be tapering.
4. Make a large horizontal incision at your waist.
5. Stick your hand in and pull out your intestines and bowels.
6. Snip off nose and ears.
7. Stretch out ears with pliers and staple them to the top of your head
8. Use garden shears to remove lower jaw.

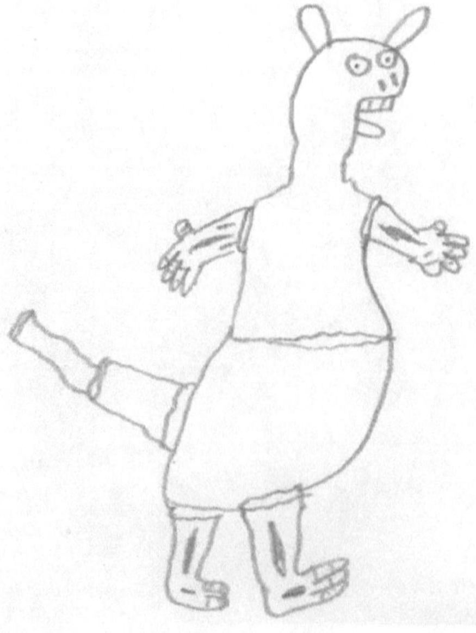

## Kinkajou

1. Use razor blades to slice out eye lids.
2. Rub black dye into eye balls.
3. Stretch out ears with pliers.
4. Sew up mouth.
5. Slice off nose and glue onto your mouth.
6. Remove the skin and flesh from your fingers and thumbs at the second knuckle.
7. Cut off one leg and cut it in half at the knee.
8. Sew the upper part of the leg to the bottom of your back and the lower back onto the leg used to be.

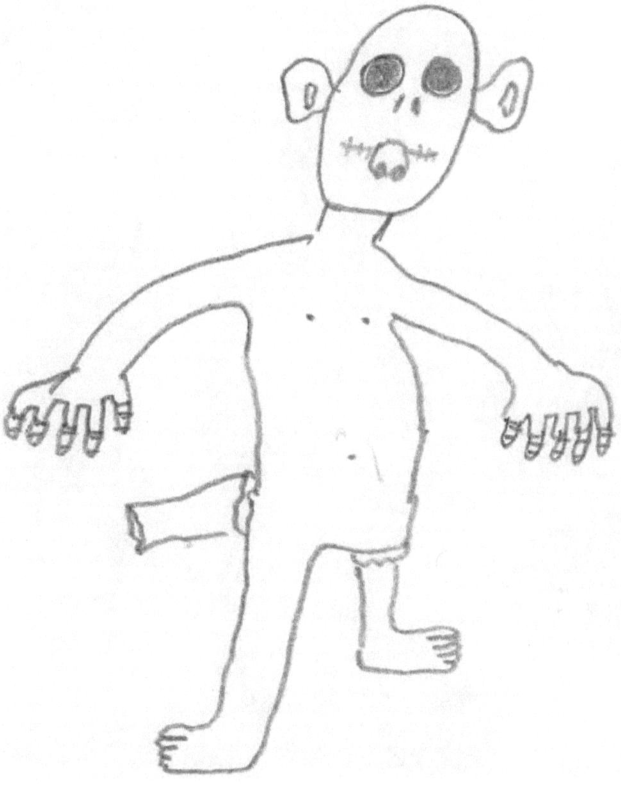

## Koala

1. Chub up by spending a week eating duck grease.
2. Amputate legs at the knee.
3. Cut off the feet. Snip off the toes and staple the feet to the sides of your head. Snip off original ears.
4. Sew an oval shaped patch of black leather to your face so it covers your nose and mouth.
5. Chisel away at the bone around your eyes so that the sockets collapse in on themselves.
6. Cut off fingers at the second knuckle.

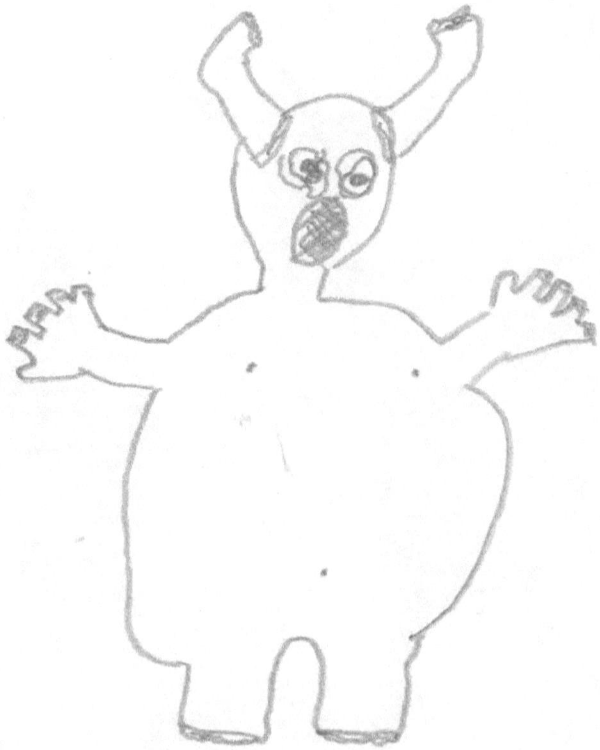

## Leopard

It's a spotted tiger dude.

## Lion

Replicate Tiger procedure. Remove all pubic hair and glue to your neck to make a mane. If you do not have enough pubic hair borrow a friends. (Do not give back.)

## Llama

1. Amputate feet and hands.
2. Slice off all the flesh and bone from your lower legs.
3. Do the same to your arms.
4. Grab your head with both hands, break your neck and push gently but firmly. Keep pushing till your neck begins to stretch out and your spine starts to exit through your neck hole. Continue this till the spine is almost completely out of the neck.
5. Cover the exposed spine in paper mache.
6. Lightly prolapse rectum.

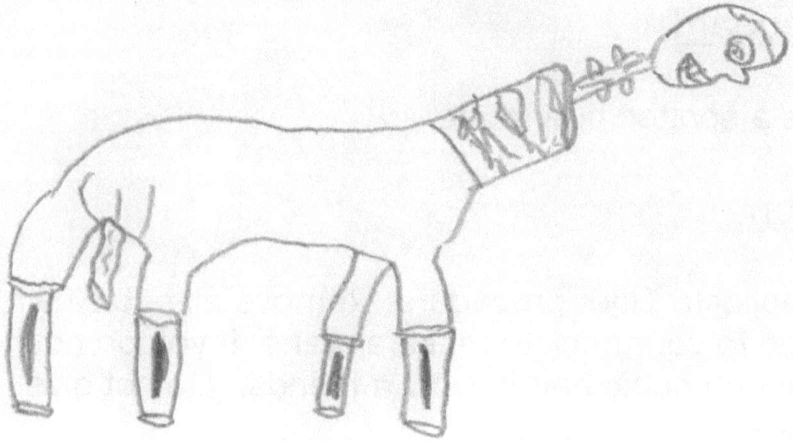

Lynx

Replicate Cat procedure. Stretch arms. Make ears longer and sharper.

Mandrill

Replicate Baboon procedure. Paint face red and blue.

Meerkat

1. Starve yourself till you look fairly skeletal.
2. Place a metal bowl on your head and hit it all over with a hammer. Do this for 2 nights straight. Now remove the bowl and behold your new head shape.
3. Stick your face in a vacuum cleaner till it tapers.
4. Sew your upper arms to your sides.
5. Mangle feet with a mallet. Then knead the flesh and bone together.

6. Amputate legs at the knee.
7. Cut off feet and stick two sticks inside them. Jam them back into the still attached upper legs.
8. Sew the lower legs together and staple them to your lower back.

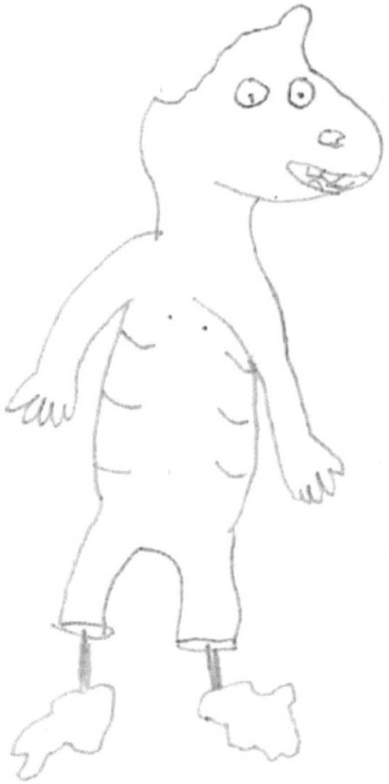

## Mongoose

(see Meerkat.)

## Moose

1. Slice open your torso and remove all your ribs. They will be firmly embedded into your skeletal system so use a nut cracker to snap them off.

2. Glue all your right side ribs together so that they all jut out. Do the same to the left side ribs.
3. Glue these "antlers" into the top of your skull.
4. Use an electric carving knife to cut out one buttock. Glue this to the end of your face.
5. Cut off your hands and feet, in that order.

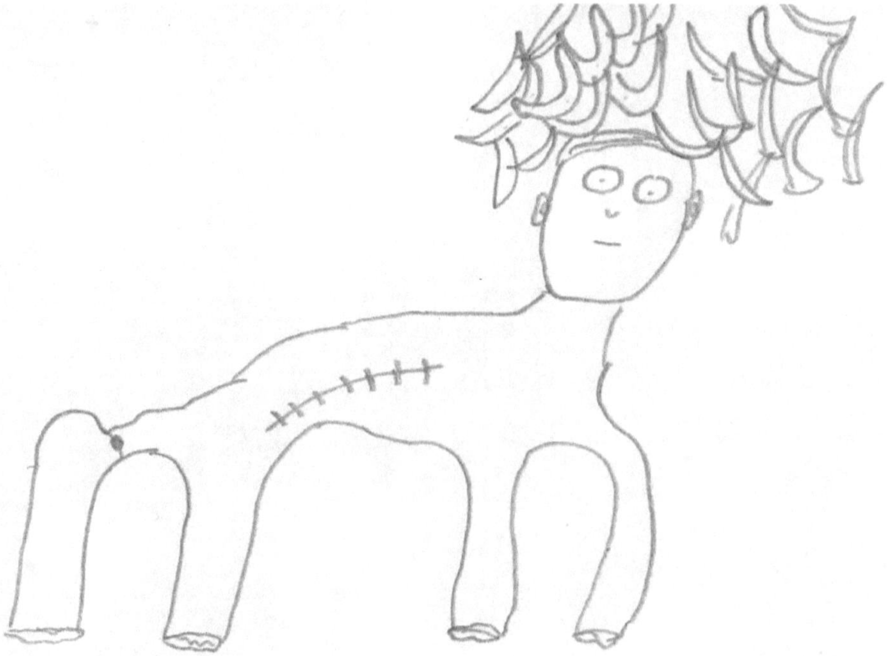

## Mouse

1. Use garden shears to cut off your head and then your neck. Disregard neck.
2. Very swiftly staple your head back onto your shoulders.
3. Use the shears again to cut off your entire lower jaw.

4. Use pliers to stretch out ears.
5. Cut off arms and legs.
6. Cut off hands and feet. Glue them back onto your shoulders and the bottom of your torso.
7. Get a butter knife. Wedge it into your spine and gently pull so that you disconnect the entire spine in one piece from the body.
8. Insert the spine into your anus.
9. Use spray paint to permanently blacken your eye balls.
10. Glue two dozen fine pubic hairs to your face. These are your whiskers.

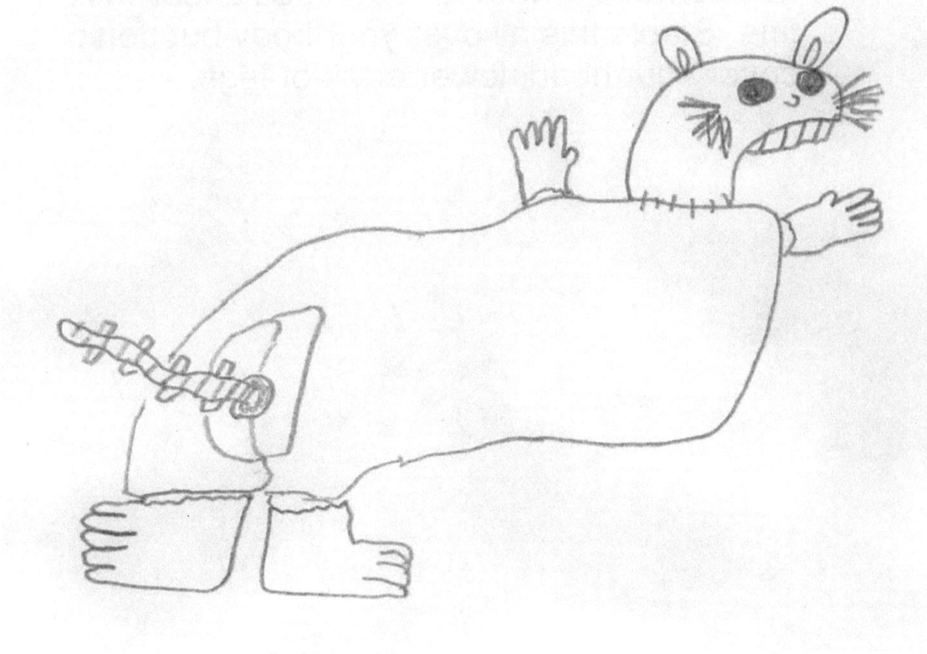

## Musk-ox

1. Slice open your chest with a scalpel or bit of broken bottle.
2. Use a hammer to break two of your ribs. Snap them off.

3. Stab these two ribs violently into the sides of your head till they get stuck.
4. Use a hot iron to completely burn off your nose and lips.
5. Sew up your mouth.
6. Glue your chin to the bottom of your neck.
7. Remove your scalp.
8. Cut off your hands and feet.
9. Get a sheet or rug. It would be preferable to use something with fur but a bed sheet will be fine. Staple this all over your body but don't cover your head, lower arms or legs.

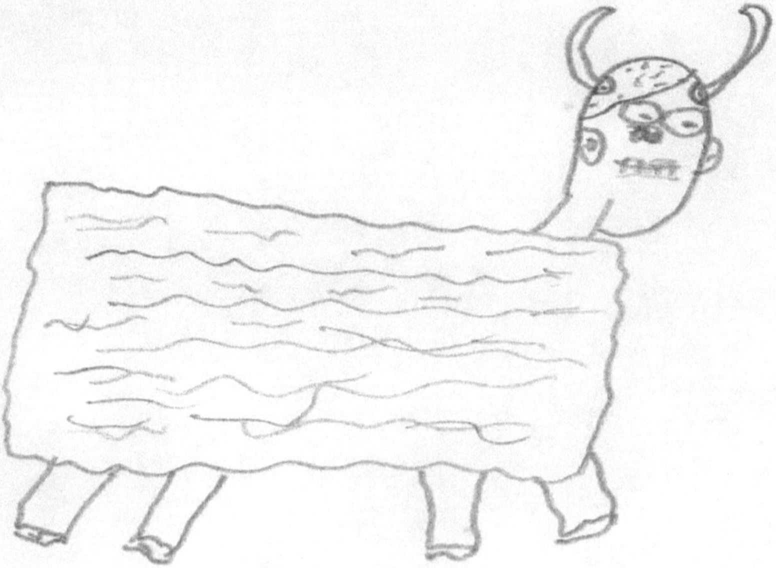

## Mole rat

You really wanna be a mole rat dude? SERIOUSLY?!

Urgh, fine. Replicate Mouse procedure. Remove all your hair. I can't believe you made me look up pictures of mole rats. I'm not getting paid enough for this book. Do you know how little royalties I actually get for this? That is if anyone will even print it.

## Ocelot

Conversely it was lovely looking at pictures of these beautiful creatures.

Replicate Cat procedure. Give yourself Tiger markings.

## Opossum

1. Snip off ears.
2. Remove your scrotum. Cut into two ovals. Staple to the top of your head. If you do not own a scrotum acquire one or use your labe.
3. Smack yourself in the face with a mallet repeatedly. Do this till it is pretty much mush.
4. Now you can mold this mush to your liking. In this case you want to shape the face so that it tapers at the end. Basically make it the rough approximation of a cone.
5. Amputate your legs and the arms at the knee and elbow.
6. Cut the fingers off your severed hands.
7. Glue your fingers to your arm stumps.
8. Skin one of your severed legs. Roll the skin up into a tube. Blow a bit of air into it then seal.
9. Staple this to your lower back.

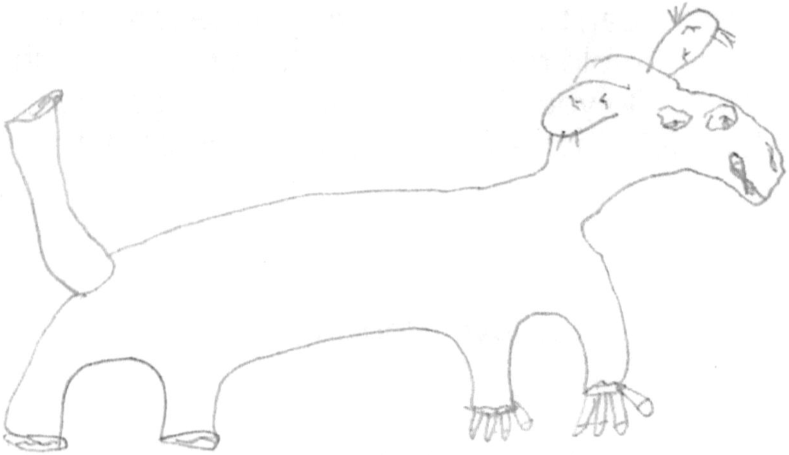

## Orangutan

Replicate Orangutan procedure. Dye fur ginger. Inject forehead with a mixture of half water half grit blended together.

## Pig

1. Amputate legs and arms at the knee and elbow.
2. Remove all hair from head and body.
3. Use pliers to stretch your ears out as far as you can.
4. Flatten nose with a mallet.
5. Use a syringe to suck the fluid out of your eyes.
6. Cut off your lower jaw with garden shears.
7. Cut the tips off your thumbs and four fingers. Glue these to your arm stumps..

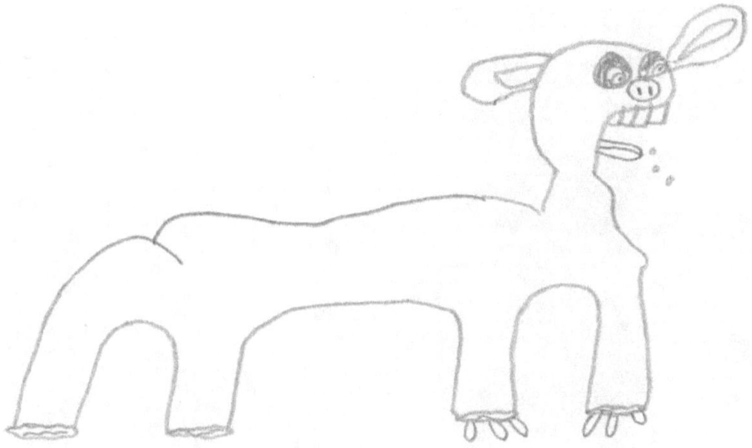

## Porcupine

1. Go into the woods and bring back two thousand sticks. You can visit the woods multiple times rather than collect all the sticks in one trip. They should be thin, average length and unmoist.
2. Use a sharp knife to whittle the sticks into thin sharp points.
3. Stab these all over your body. Aim to have one fifth of the stick penetrating inside your body. This generally is enough to stay in and still look nice.
4. Cut out your lower jaw with an electric carving knife.
5. Amputate your arms and legs at the elbow and knee. **[I just realized how many times I've written this in the book. It's quite a recurring instruction.]**
6. Staple one of your amputated legs to your anus.

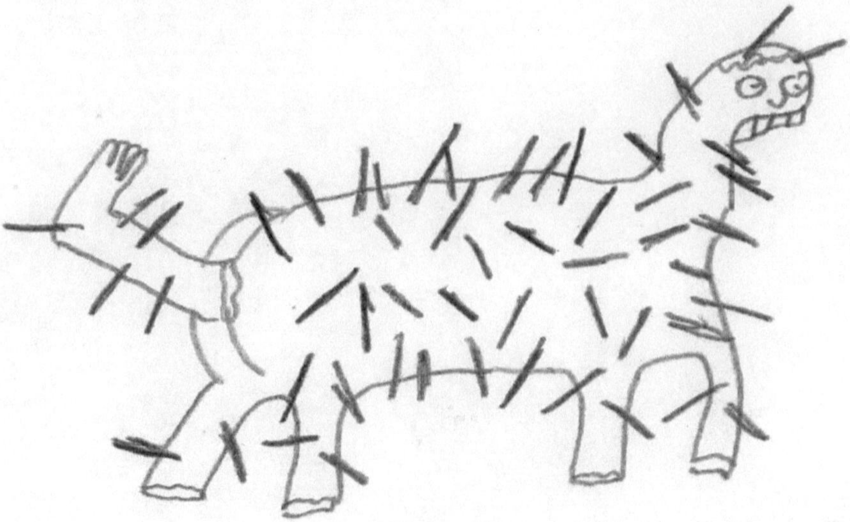

## Possum

See Opossum. Don't argue with me. They're the same creature and you know it!

## Prarie dog

1. Stick your head in the axle of a moving car or motorbike tire. Do this for about 45 seconds.
2. Sew your upper arms to your sides.
3. Cut off your legs.
4. Cut the feet off the amputated legs and glue to the bottom of your torso.
5. Crudely slice off a bit of flesh from your severed leg. Nail this to your lower back.

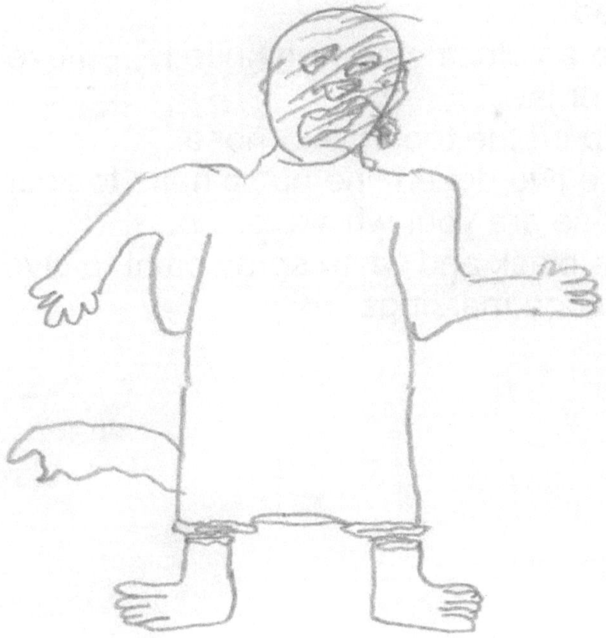

## Rat

Replicate Mouse procedure. Make tail longer. Get filthy. Rats are filthy. Yeah, I said it.

## Racoon

1. Amputate arms and legs.
2. Cut off hands and feet and glue them back onto your body.
3. Smack your head into a wall till your neck disappears.
4. Staple a severed leg to the bottom of your back.

5. Snip off ears and glue them to the top of your head.
6. Use an electric carving knife to remove your lower jaw.
7. Snip off the top of your nose.
8. Glue two dozen fine pubic hairs to your face. These are your whiskers.
9. Use black and white spray paint to give yourself raccoon markings.

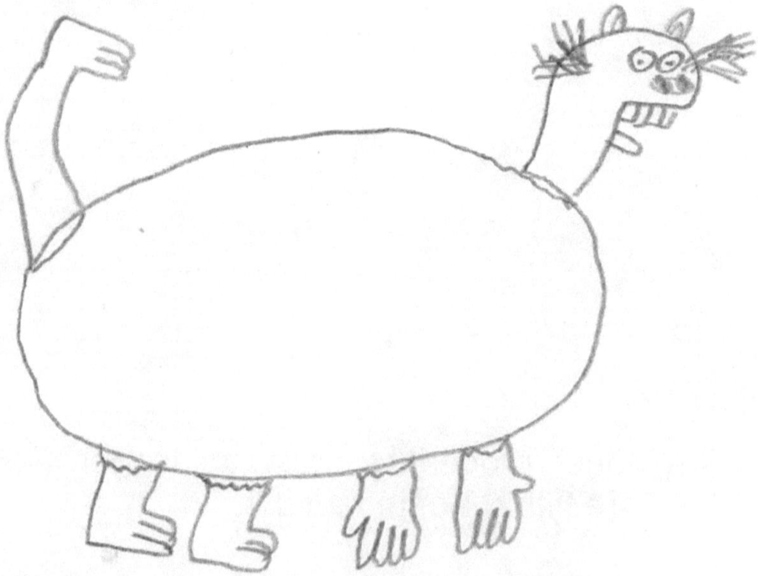

## Skunk

Do the Racoon Procedure. Be a smelly bastard. I know the two look nothing alike but I wrote an entire procedure for Skunk then realized it was exactly the same as the Racoon one. Trust me, you'll look like a skunk.

## Sloth

1. Cut off your arms and legs.
2. Sew your arms where your legs used to be and vice versa.
3. Snip off the end of your nose.
4. Cut off your lips.
5. Cut off all the skin around your neck. Stretch it out so it is as wide as your shoulders then glue it back on.
6. Cut out your eye lids with a razor blade.
7. Cut off your hands and feet.
8. Snip off six fingers (or four if you want to be a two toed sloth) and glue them to your leg stumps.

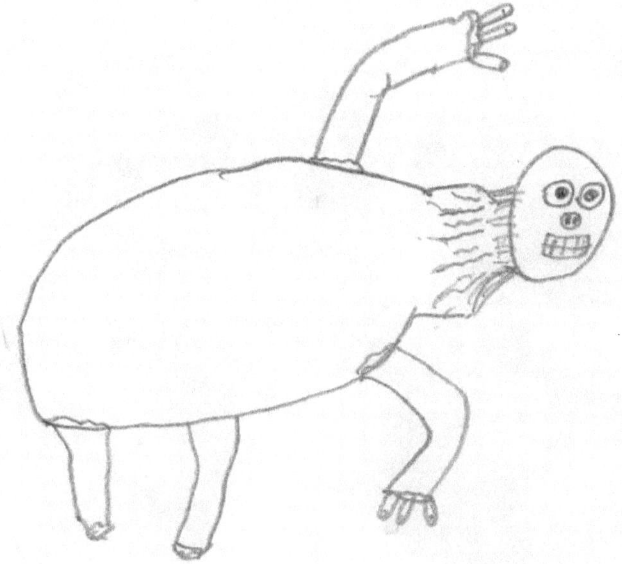

## Squirrel

(See chipmunk.)

## Tapir

1. Grab your jaws with both hands and snap them open.
2. Amputate your arms and legs at the knee and elbow.
3. Cut the foot off one of the legs.
4. Staple this leg to your nose.
5. Use pliers to stretch out your ears.
6. Cut out your eye lids with a razor blade.

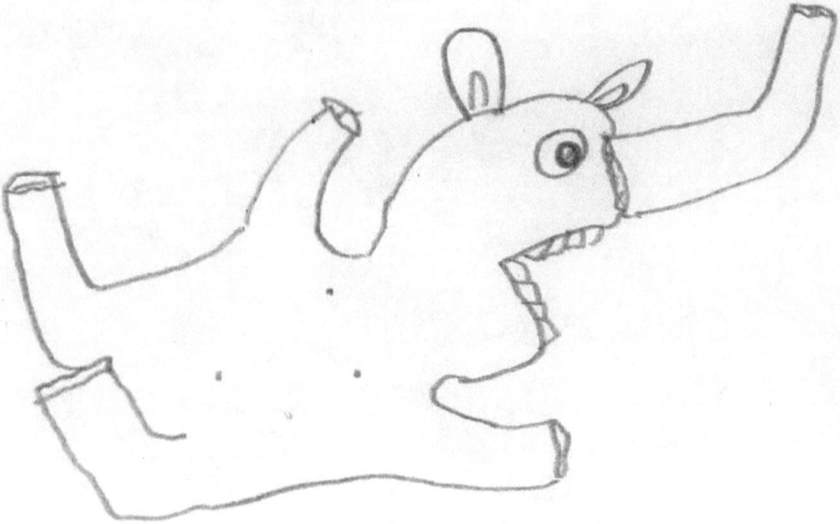

## Tasmanian Devil

This is instructions to look like the real life creature. Not the cartoon character. Sorry.

1. Amputate arms and legs at the knee and elbow. **[God I'm sick of saying that. Damn mammals with their stupid short stumpy FUCKING legs.]**
2. Use garden shears to remove your lower jaw.
3. Cut off the middle fingers from the severed hands. Use a knife to remove the flesh off them and sharpen them to points.
4. Jam these fingers into your gums.
5. Stretch out your ears with pliers.
6. Cut off your nose.
7. Glue two dozen fine pubic hairs to your face.

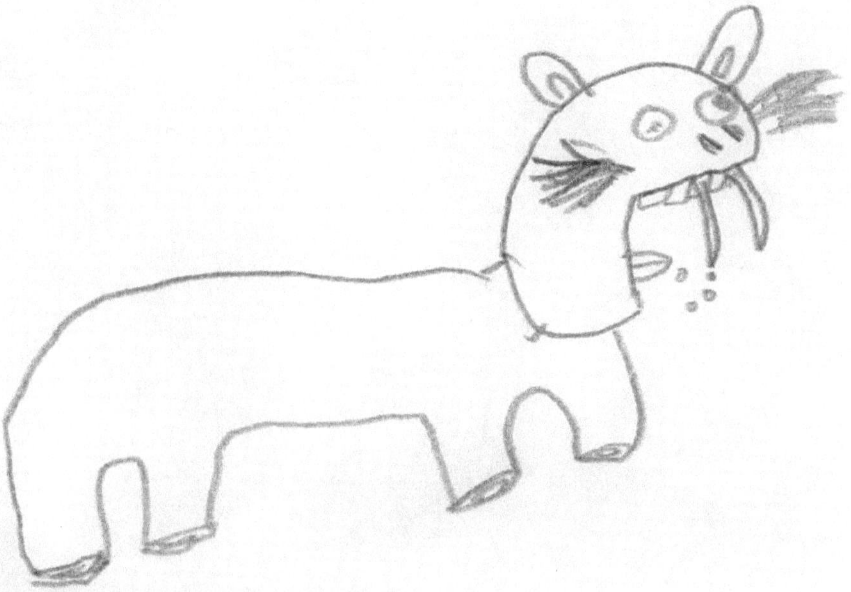

## Tiger

1. Cut off fingers at the second knuckle. Use a knife to remove the skin off the rest of the fingers and sharpen them into points.
2. Cut off toes.
3. Flatten nose with a hammer.
4. Pull out your upper and lower canine teeth.
5. Cut off lips and glue mouth closed.
6. Glue lips to your chin and your canine teeth to the lips.
7. Cut off ears and staple them to the top of your head.
8. Procure a knife that could be used for removing limpets from rocks. Use it against each of your vertebrae one by one and snag them out of your back. Do this till you have disconnected your entire spine. It should still be intact. If not, oh dear.
9. Jam the spine into your anus.

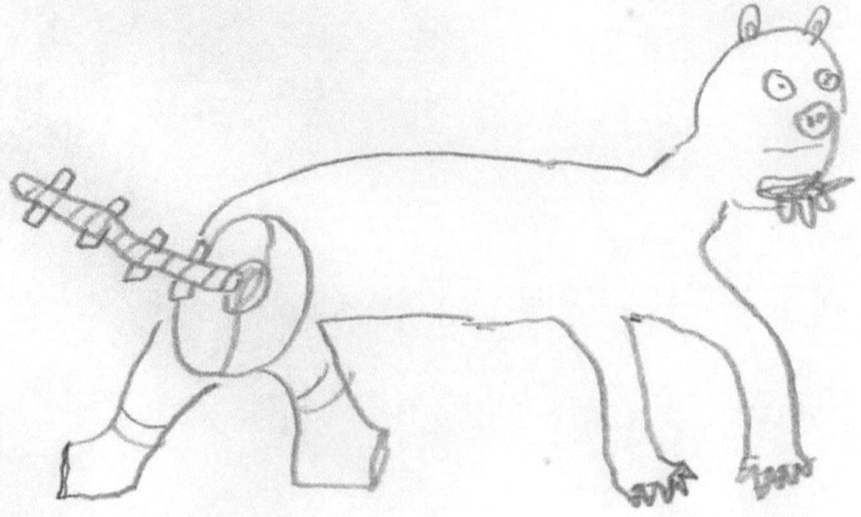

## Wallaby

Replicate Kangaroo procedure. Use a microwave to compress yourself.

## Warthog

1. Cut off hands and feet.
2. Make a horizontal incision at the top of your back. Wedge a shoe horn or crow bar into your shoulder blades and snap them out.
3. Solder your shoulder blades to the sides of your face.
4. Make a horizontal incision on your chest. Use a hammer to snap off two ribs and pull them out.
5. Jam the ribs into your cheeks. Use hammer to embed them.
6. Cut off nose, flatten it with a rolling pin and glue it to your chin.
7. Cut off ears, stretch with pliers and staple them to the top of your head.
8. Scalp yourself, roll the scalp up into a tube and staple it your anus.
9. Glue several pubic tufts to your scalp.

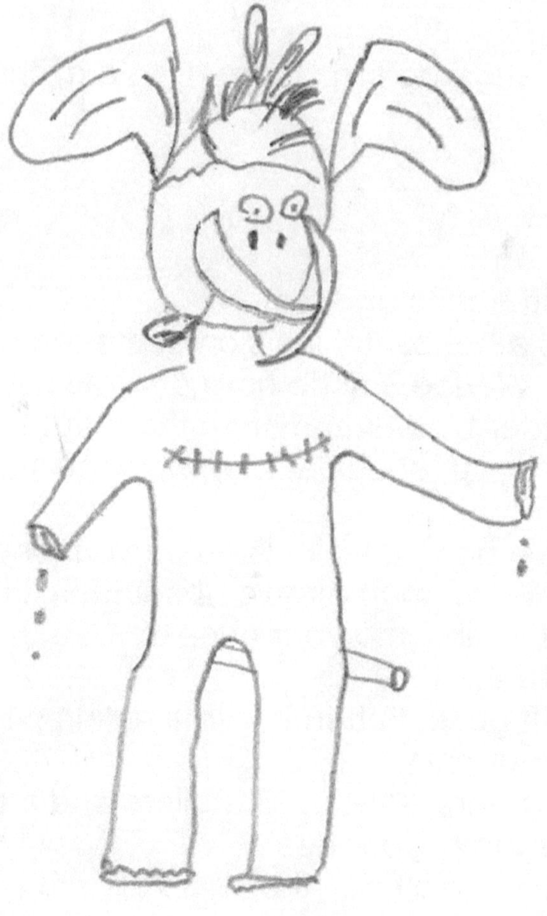

Water Buffalo

1. Amputate arms and legs at the knee and elbow.
2. Use a knife to cleave the skin and flesh off the arms legs.
3. Solder the arm bones to your temples.
4. Snap the wrist bones so that the hands are at a 90 degree angle.

5. Staple one of the severed legs to your lower back
6. Use pliers to stretch out ears as far as you can.
7. Glue mouth closed.
8. Cut off nose and glue it to your chin.

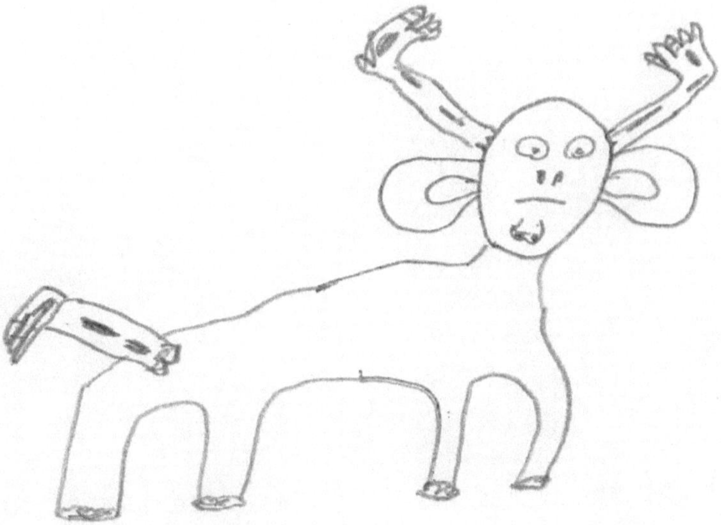

## Wolf

(See dog. Be more aggressive.)

## Wolverine

1. Grab your upper and lower jaws with both hands. Pull hard to snap the jaws. Open them as wide as you can and pull again to stretch them out.

2. Use a hammer and chisel to sharpen your teeth into points.
3. Snip off your nose.
4. Amputate arms and legs at the elbow and knee.
5. Cut hands and feet off and staple them back onto body.
6. Cleave the skin off your fingers and toes. Sharpen them into points.
7. Remove spine.

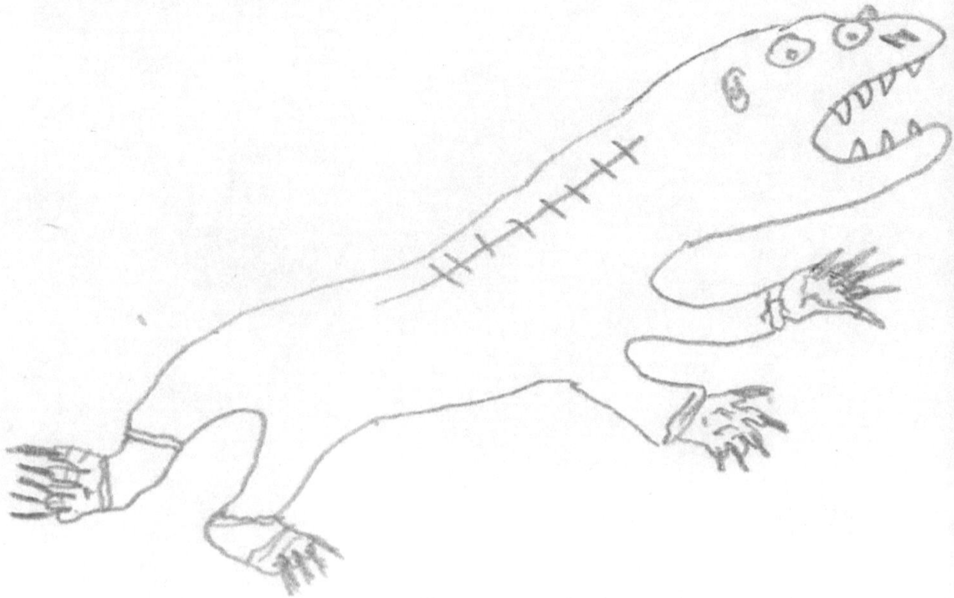

## <u>Zebra</u>

It’s a fucking stripey horse. I’m not being lazy by referring you to another procedure. Get off my back!

# Section 2: Birds

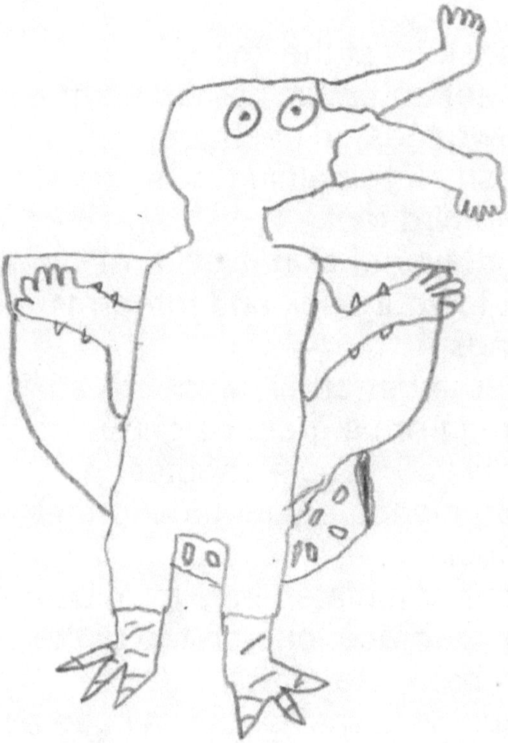

Birds come in a vast variety of sizes and colours. But they all share a basic shape. Follow these steps to attain the basic body type of a bird. Then amputate or elongate the parts of your body that match your desires bird. Finally spray paint your body the desired colour.

For this procedure you need to procure a layer of skin the height and width of your body. I know this is easier said than done but don't worry – it is perfectly fine to collect smaller pieces of skin and patch them together.

1. Amputate legs at the knees.
2. Cut off feet and attach to leg stumps.
3. Cut off two toes on each foot.
4. Slice flesh off remaining toes and shape the bone into bird feet.
5. Get your layer of skin. Now turn it sideways and staple it to your back and forearms. These are your wings.
6. Sew your upper arms to your torso.
7. Now hang from a great height using only your teeth until your face elongates.
8. If needed elongate your face further with a heavy door.
9. Take your amputated legs from before and sew them to your face, one on top of the other to create a beak like effect.
10. Finally, to make your tail use a plunger to collapse your anus in on itself.
11. Remove teeth with hammer and use them to decorate your new tail.

Modification Tips:

**Chicken**: Staple hands to the end of your rectum. Remove scrotum and staple to chin. Bash head against a wall.
**Duck**: Staple the leg jaws together. Remove spine.
**Pelican**: Remove all the bones from lower leg jaw.
**Penguin**: Glue upper arms to sides. Cut off half of leg jaws and sharpen the ends of them.
**Parrot**: Cut off most of your leg jaws. Cleave off the flesh and sharpen the bone.
**Turkey**: Use hot iron to flatten out and stretch rectum till it resembles a semi-circle. Remove scrotum and staple to chin. Burn face with a blow torch.

# Section 3: Reptiles

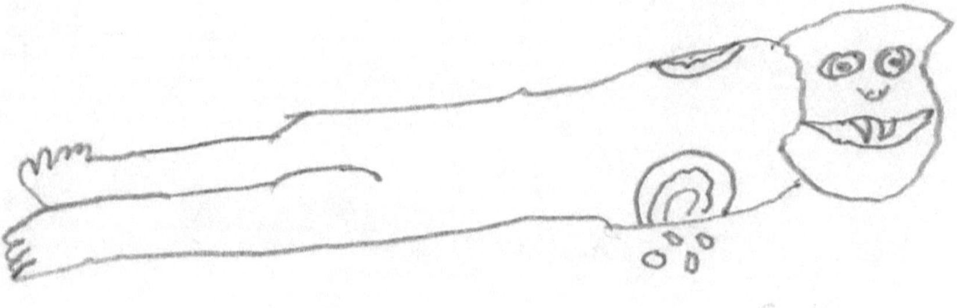

To become a reptile you need that distinctive dry scaly skin. This is where sand paper comes in handy. Rub the paper all over your body till it attains a reptilian texture. Add colour and markings to skin where needed. This must be done before performing all reptile Transformations.

## Alligator

1. Remove teeth and sharpen them into fangs.
2. Cut off feet and sew them together at the wounds. This will be your new alligator mouth
3. Glue the fangs to the inside of the feet.
4. Staple the feet to your face. You look ferocious already!
5. Cut off feet at the knees. Sew these together. This is your new tail.
6. Sew the tail to your anus.

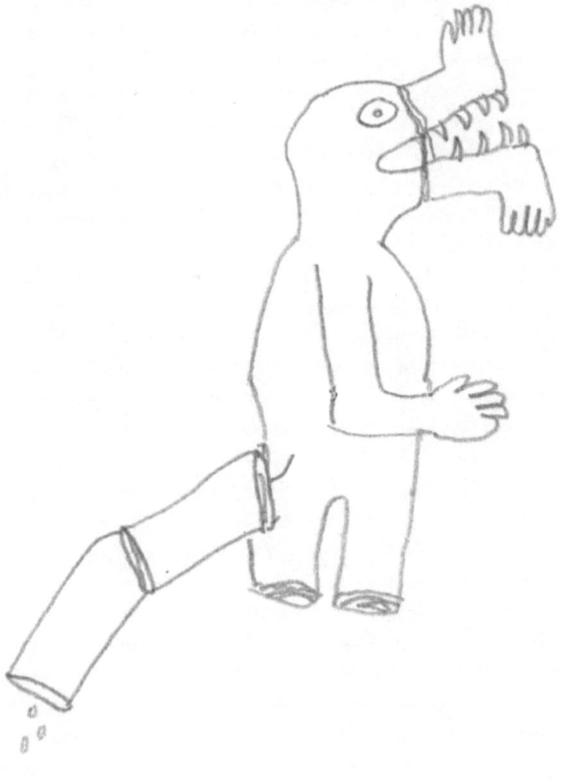

## Crocodile

(See alligator. Let's be honest, the scientific community all agree that there is literally NO difference between alligators and crocodiles.)

## Lizard

1. Follow instructions number 5 and 6 of the Alligator procedure.
2. Cut off nose and ears.
3. Use a vice to make your face sharper and less wide.
4. Replace your feet with your hands and your hands with your feet.

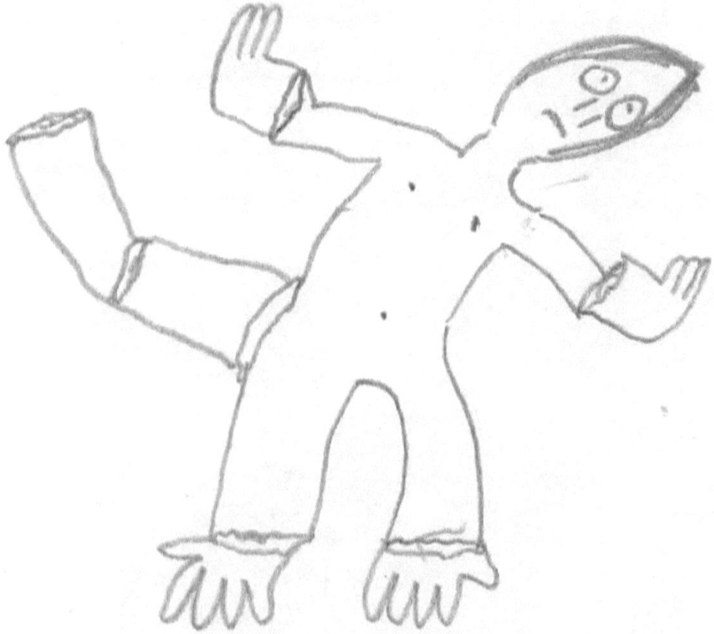

## Snake

1. Sew the insides of your legs together so it appears you have one massive leg.
2. To attain a snake like face go with the traditional method of smacking your head against a large rock.
3. Knock out all but two teeth. Sharpen these into fangs.
4. Slice the sides of your mouth open.
5. Remove all your ribs and leg bones to give yourself a slender, slithery body.
6. Finally position a power saw and cut off both your arms completely. Cauterize wounds IMMEDIATELY.

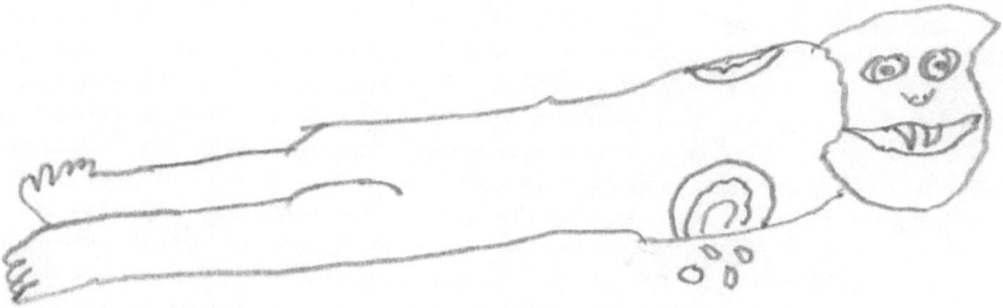

## Turtle

Before starting the procedure construct yourself a realistic, roomy and comfortable turtle shell. This can be done out of any material you see fit.

1. Fuse turtle shell to back.
2. Cut off nose and ears.

3. Remove all skin and flesh from face.
4. Remove neck bones.
5. Elongate neck.
6. Amputate forearms and lower legs.

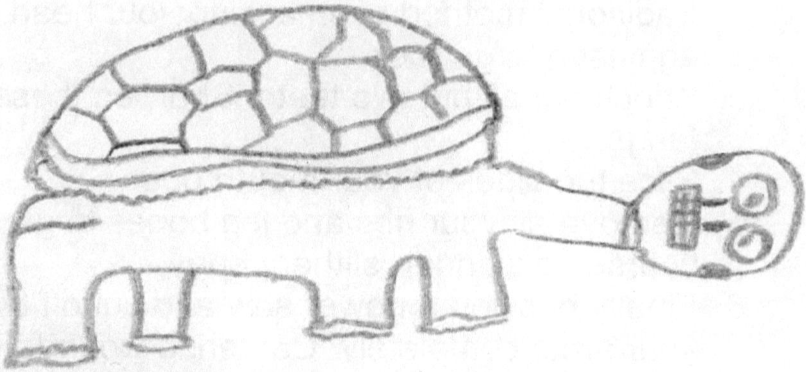

# Section 4: Amphibians

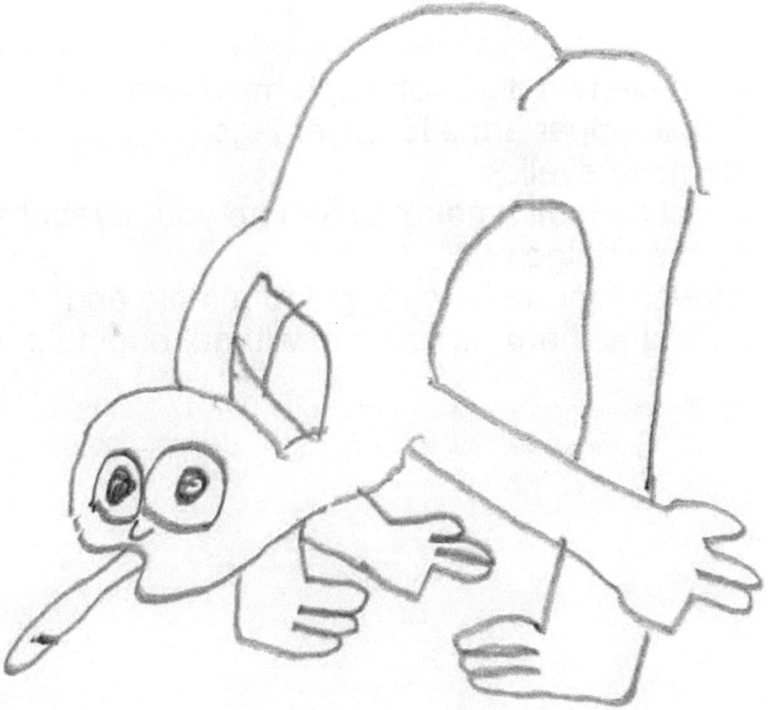

For each of these procedures you need to remove your ears and nose. You must also replicate the skin texture technique talked about in the Reptile section. Unlike a reptile you also need to have moist skin. For this use the sand paper to remove ALL skin, leaving a layer of exposed gooey flesh. You can either paint this green or wait for it to become infected.

## Frog

1. Remove two digits off each hand and foot.
2. Staple upper arms to upper legs.
3. Remove eyelids.
4. Inject a small amount of air into your eyeballs so they bulge out.
5. Stretch tongue by nailing it to a table and pulling as hard as you can without ripping it off.

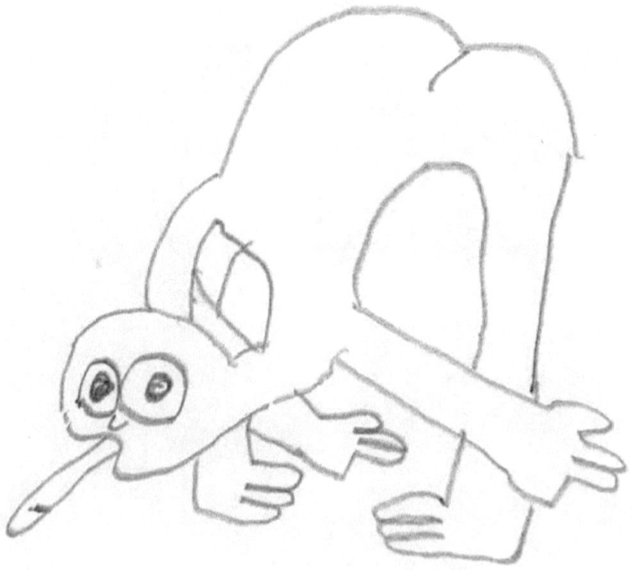

The reader – “My God, he just used the same picture for 2 page sides. Can he do that?!”

## Newt

1. Repeat all steps of the Frog technique EXCEPT step 2.
2. Follow the instructions for making your own tail in the Alligator procedure in the Reptile section.

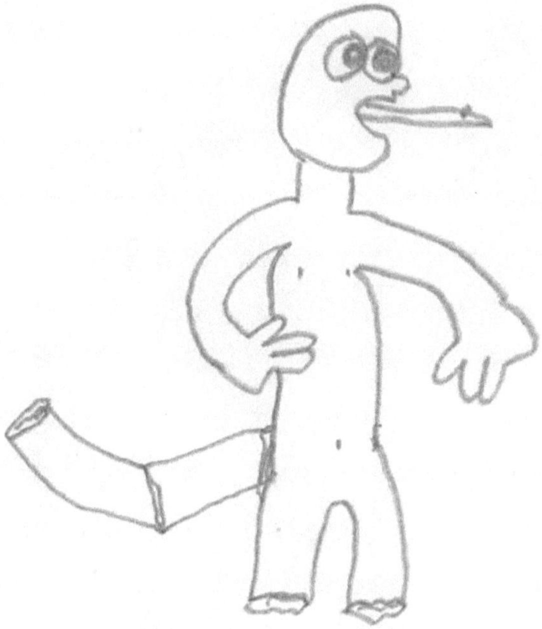

## Salamander

If there’s a noticeable difference between a salamander and a newt I don’t wanna hear about it.

## Toad

Follow the instructions for toad and become morbidly obese.

Blimey that was a short section wasn't it?

# Section 5: Marine Animals

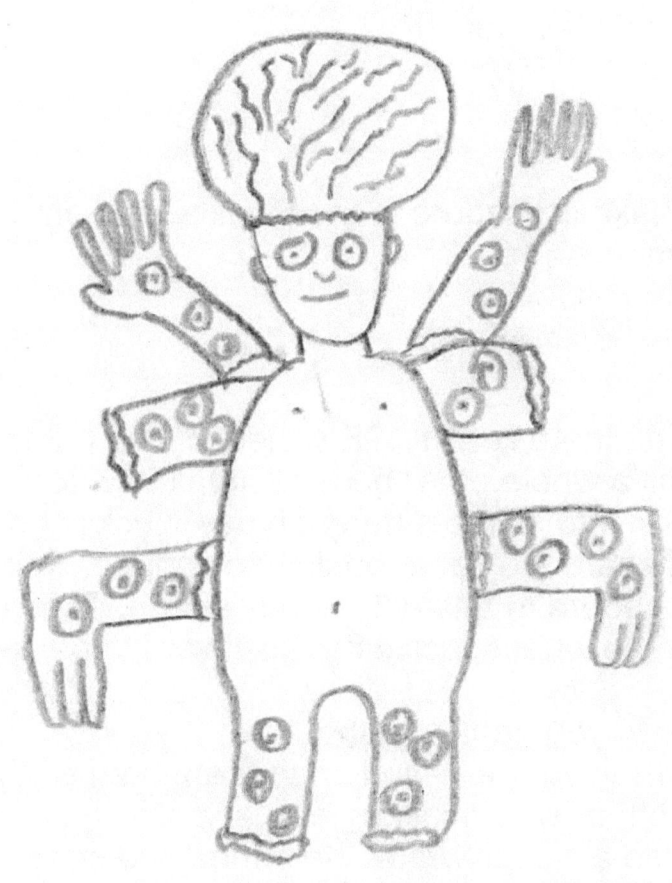

## Dolphin

Replicate the Orca procedure (found below) with these changes:

- Do not chub up.
- Dive into a bath tub full of light blue paint rather than black tar.

## Eel

[See Snake procedure in the Reptile Section. Cover self in mucus.]

## Fish

Like birds there is a HUGE variety of fish out there. It would fill a whole other book to detail how to transform into all the different types. Luckily however they all share the same basic body shape. Replicate this procedure to attain this body shape. Then modify it based on what specific fish you want to be.

1. Sew your legs together.
2. Break your feet and snap them both so they are both at a vertical angle.
3. Use a vice to break the bones and soften the flesh in your feet.
4. Use vice to crush head inwards so it has virtually no width.

5. Cut off one arm. Slice it into three pieces – hand, forearm and upper arm.
6. Staple the hand to your back. This is now a fin!
7. Dispose of the other two arm sections.
8. Sew your still attached upper arm to your stomach.

Modification tip – If you want to be a swordfish simply remove your spine and jam into your nose.

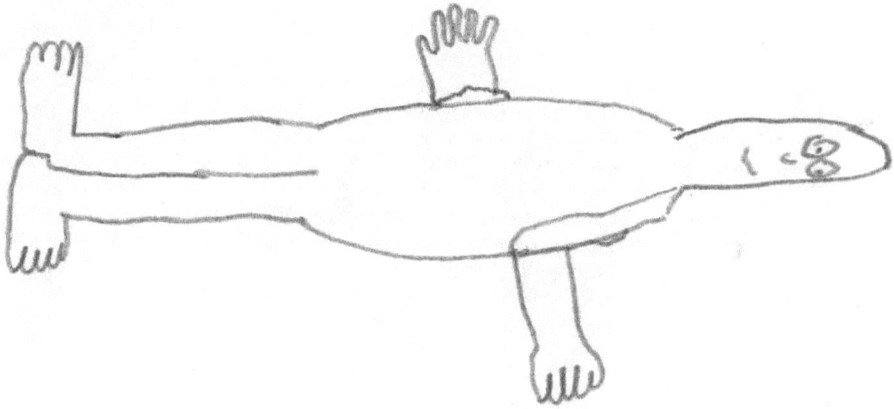

## Manatee

1. Cut off arms at the elbow.
2. Now crush your still attached upper arms with a mallet.
3. Slice open your legs and use a pin hammer to break all the bones inside.
4. When the bones have been broken pull them all out and seal up the legs.
5. Do the same thing to your feet.
6. Tear off your genitals with your bare hands.
7. Shave all the hair off your body.

8. This instruction must be done as quickly as possible in order to prevent death:
9. Use garden shears to decapitate self at the base of the neck.
10. Now cut head in half at the jaw.
11. Swiftly glue the top part of the head back onto the neck stump.

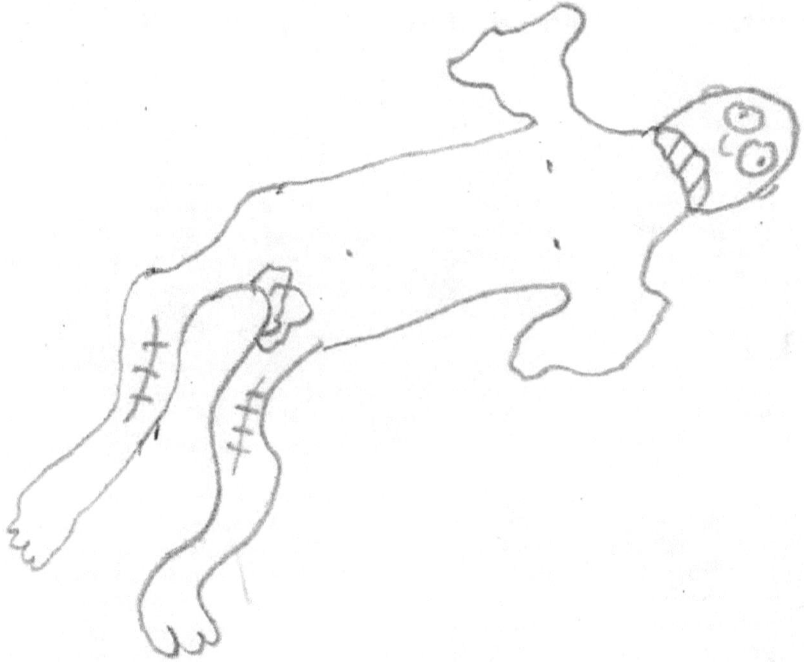

## Manta Ray

1. Chisel out your entire spine.
2. Now use a scalpel to remove all your skin.
3. Patch the skin into one piece then fold it in half. Staple closed all but one side of the skin piece. It should look like a bed sheet made out of skin.

4. Glue the disconnected spine to one end of the skin sheet.
5. Get the chisel out again and begin the long and arduous process of removing all your bones.
6. When you have no more bones left slither into the skin sheet staple it closed from the inside.

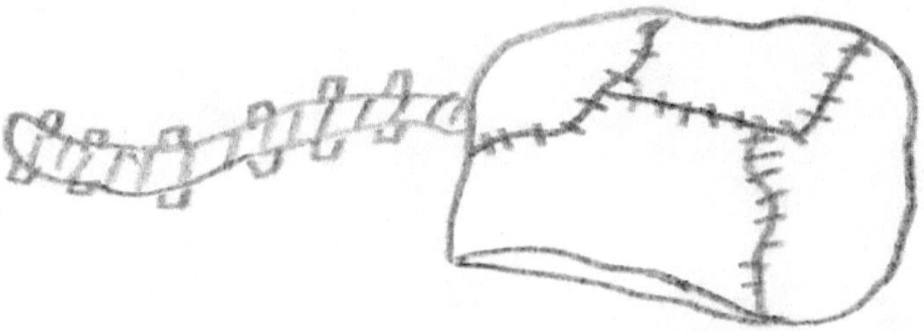

## Octopus

1. Cut off hands and feet.
2. Amputate arms and legs at the elbow and knee.
3. Glue your severed legs to the sides of your torso.
4. Glue your severed arms to your shoulders.
5. Go to a public swimming pool and rub yourself along the surfaces till you develop a verruca. Nurture and care for this verruca and use it to spread verrucae all over your arms and legs.
6. Use a power saw to saw open the top of your skull, leaving your brain exposed.
7. Rub any brand of sweet chili sauce into the brain until it begins to swell up.

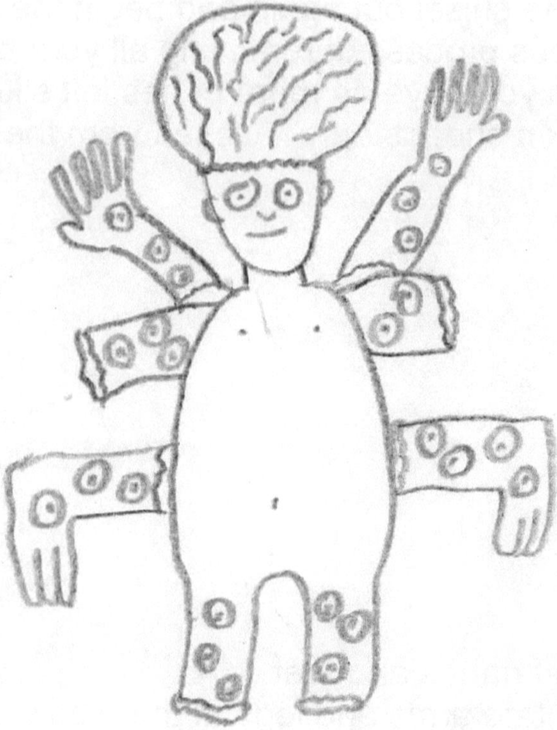

## Orca

Ah, the elegant majestic orca. This is the animal I chose to be. If you wish to perform this procedure on yourself you have great taste and you and I are kindred spirits. Perhaps one day will shall splash around together in my spacious briny bath.

1. Fuse legs and feet together with hot glue.
2. Snap feet so that they jut out sideways at a ninety degree angle.
3. Bash them with a mallet.

4. Amputate your arms at the elbow.
5. Bash the attached upper arms with a mallet.
6. Cut the hands off the amputated arms.
7. Staple one of these hands to the middle of your back.
8. Hang from a great height by your teeth until your face elongates.
9. Dive into a bath of hot tar. Wait for it to fuse onto your skin.
10. Apply white paint where necessary.
11. Chub up by slurping on your neighbour's garbage juice when in the middle of the night.

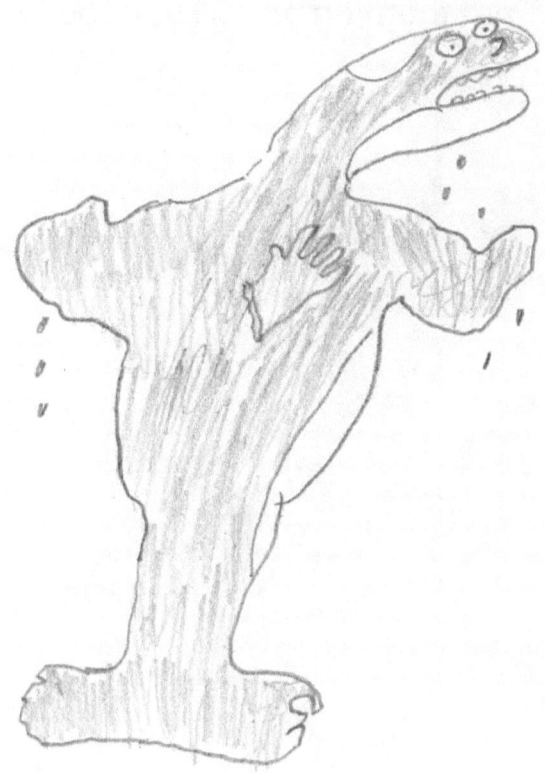

## Porpoise

Replicate Dolphin procedure. Bash face into a wall.

## Puffer fish

Replicate Fish procedure.
Remove spine. Cut vertebrae into sections and stab them all over you're your body. Use a hammer so they are properly embedded.
When you want to puff up, stick two water hoses inside yourself – one in your mouth and the other in your anus. Turn them on and fill your body to bursting point.

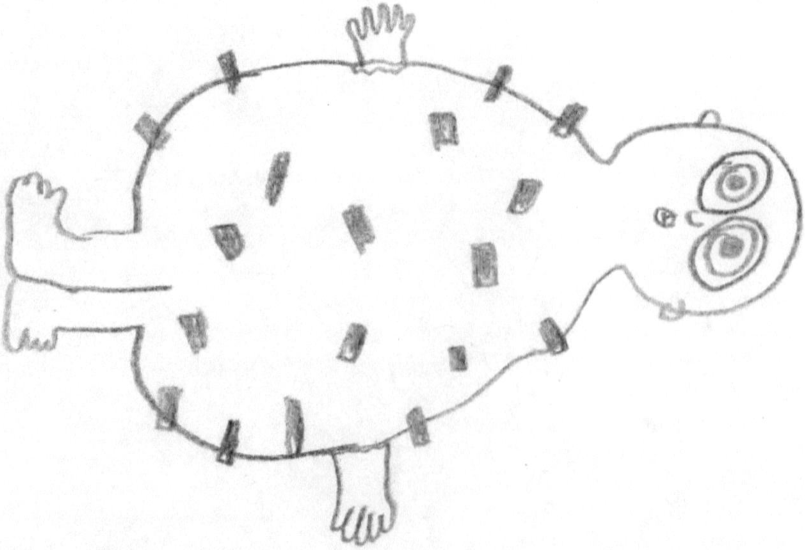

## Seal

(The animal, not the singer.)

1. Amputate arms and legs.
2. Cut off hands and feet, bash them with a mallet then reattach to body.
3. Use garden shears to remove lower jaw.
4. Make a horizontal cut on your throat, stretch the skin and staple it to your upper jaw.
5. Remove all head and body hair.
6. Slice off nose.
7. Glue a handful of pubic to your face.
8. Spend a fortnight slurping on some pudding to chub up.
9. Remove genitals.

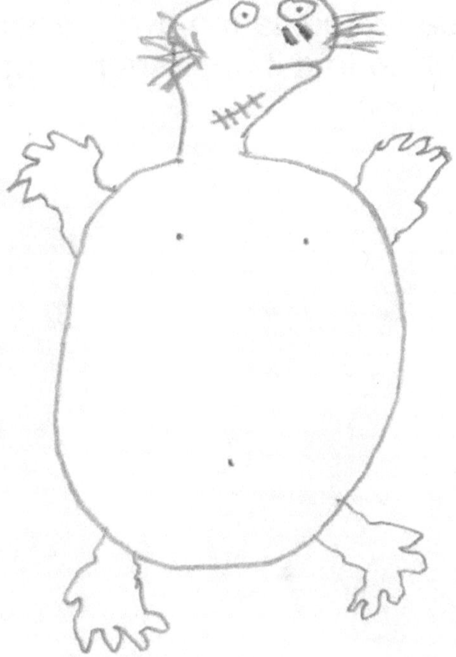

## Sea Lion

(See Seal. The animal, not the singer.)

## Shark

Replicate the Orca procedure with these changes:

- Snap the feet so they are pointing vertically rather than horizontally.
- Glue a hand to where your genitals used to be.
- Sharpen teeth
- Slice three slits into your neck. These are your gills.

If you want to be a hammer head you basically have to allow your head to be flatten by a passing car then reshape the skull so that it appears hammer-like.

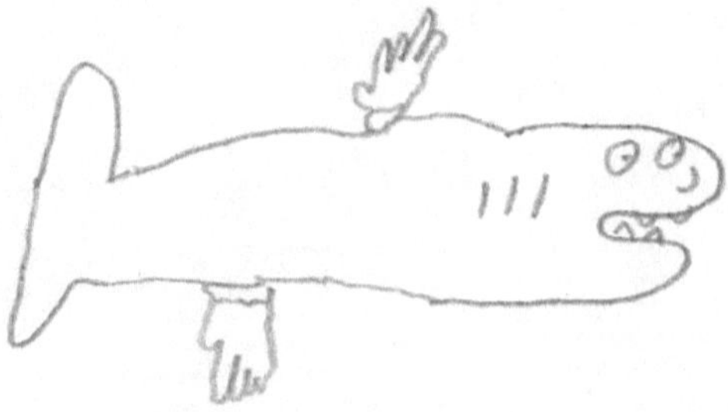

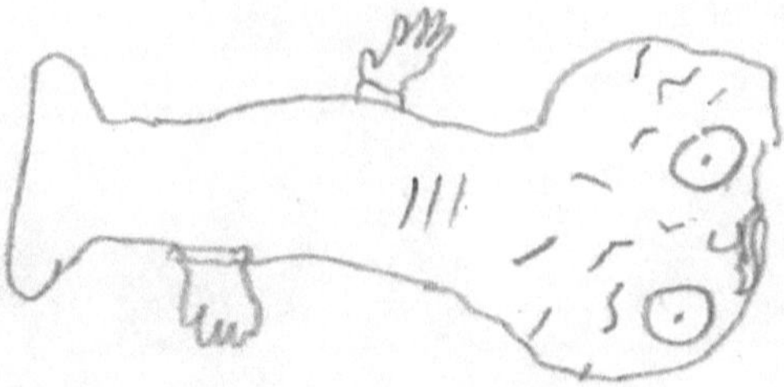

## Squid

1. Cut open legs and remove all the bone inside them.
2. Cut yourself in half at the waist.
3. Glue the leg end to the top of your head.
4. Stick your legs in a shredder for 45 seconds then pull them out again.
5. Amputate arms.
6. Remove genitals.

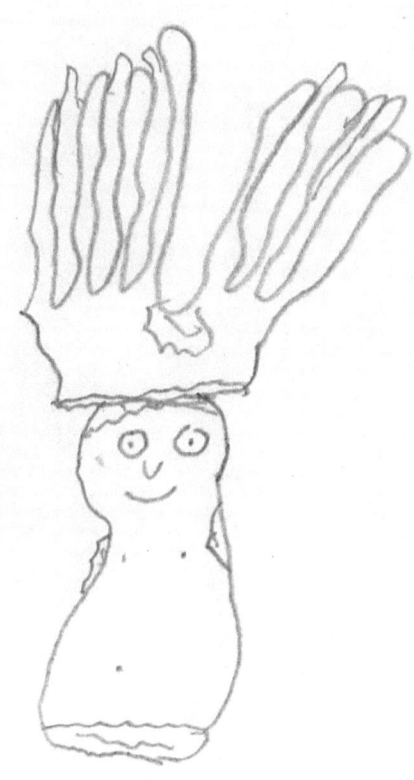

## Stingray

(See Manta Ray.)

## Whale

Replicate the Orca procedure and modify depending on what type of whale you wish to be.

This will usually entail hanging by your teeth for slightly longer to further elongate your face and slurping on more of your neighbour’s garbage juice to chub up more.

# Section 6: Land Invertebrates and Bugs

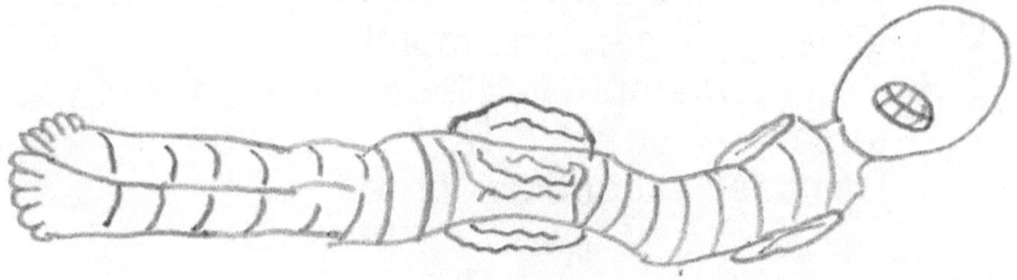

## Ant

1. Remove all the skin and flesh around your neck and space between your lower ribs and hips.
2. Use garden shears to remove lower jaw. **[How many fucking times have I written this sentence?! It's becoming SO repetitive. I may as well rename the book "How to Cut off Your Lower Jaw with Garden Shears."**
3. Amputate arms and legs at the knee and elbow. **[Goddamnit, same goes for this bloody sentence.]**
4. Cut off hands. Staple them to your temples. Glue the fingers and thumbs together.
5. Sew your amputated legs to the sides of your torso.
6. Paint self either black or red.

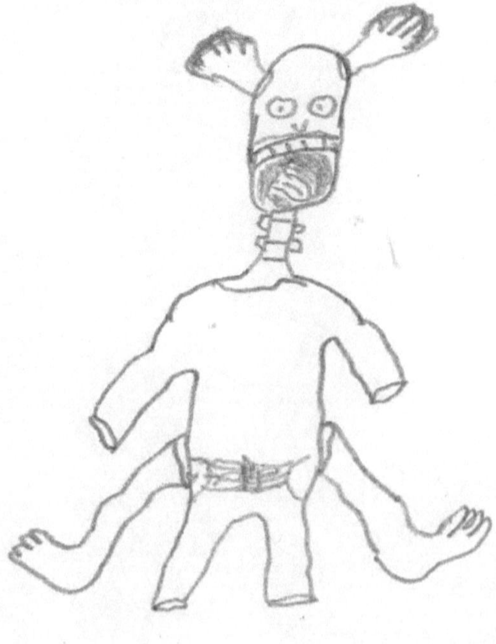

If you want to be a **Queen Ant** collapse your anus in on itself and stretch it out as far as it can without tearing.

If you want to be a **Flying Ant** slice the skin off your back, cut it into a wing shape and glue it back on.

## Bacteria

1. Modify your blender so that is powerful enough to separate single cells from eachother.
2. Dive in.

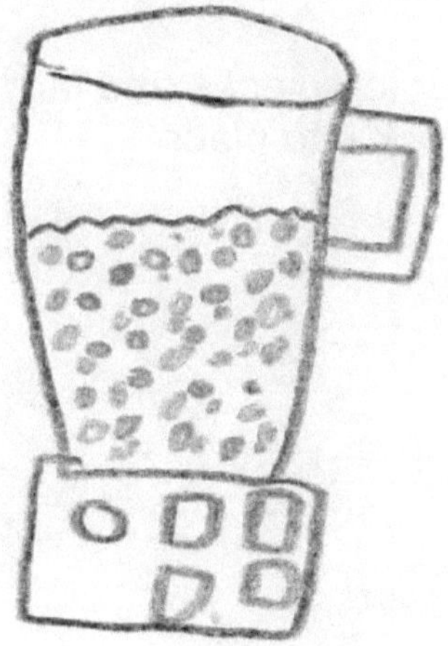

## Bee

1. First thing you'll need to do is create a pair of thin transparent wings. To do this cut a line all the way down the middle of your back. Now cut a horizontal line all the way along the bottom and top of the vertical line. Now stick both hands in the vertical cut and pull it open as wide as you can. You now have a set of rudimentary wings on your back.
   Coat the wings in glue to set them and use scissors to shape them and make them more defined.
2. Remove scalp and glue to neck.
3. Amputate both legs and cut them into four.
4. Use a hammer and chisel to chip away a small portion of the bottom of your spine. One vertebra will do. Now shape this into a sharpened point. Insert into anus with the pointy end sticking out. Voila, a stinger.
5. Spray paint body in black and yellow stripes.
6. Spray paint entire face, including eyes black.
7. Use a hammer to break four ribs, two on each side of the body. Make sure the ribs are jutting out of your torso.
8. Take your four leg pieces and jam them into the broken ribs, twist to lock into place.

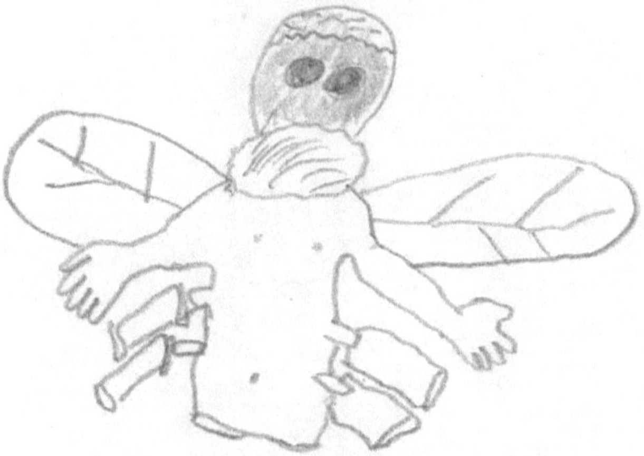

# Butterfly

1. Remove all the skin from your body. Patch the skin together into two large wing shapes. Make them as large as possible. Decorate them as you wish.
2. Amputate legs. Attach them to the top of your head.
3. Now lie on your new wings and staple each one to an upper arm.
4. Secure the wings by stapling them into your sides.

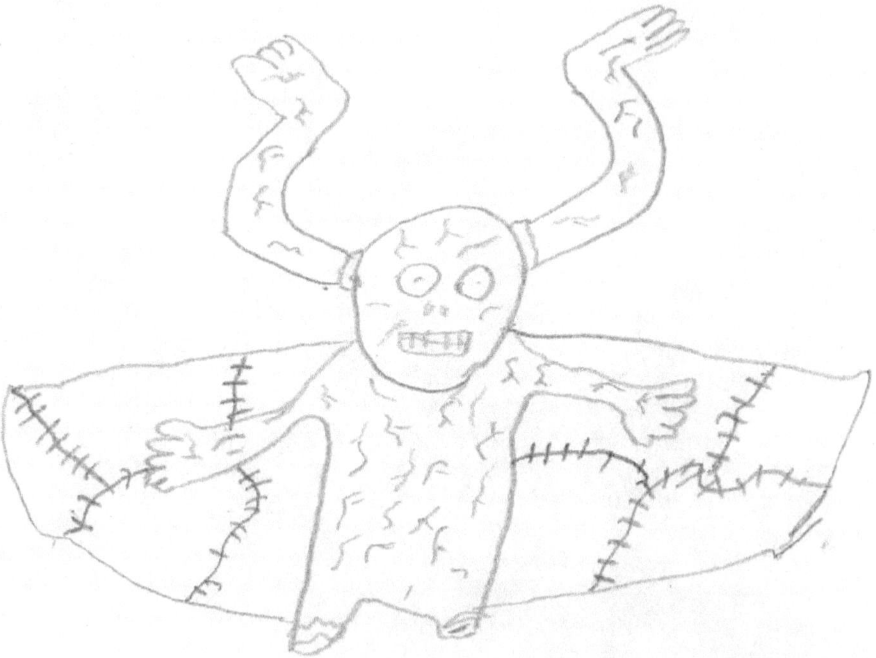

## Cicada

1. Cut a large rectangle into your back without a bottom horizontal line.
2. Peel the skin off so it is dangling from the bottom of your back.
3. Apply heat to face and body till you receive third degree burns.
4. Repeat instructions 3, 7 and 8 from the Bee procedure.
5. Use a bicycle pump to apply as a high a blood pressure as possible to your eyes.

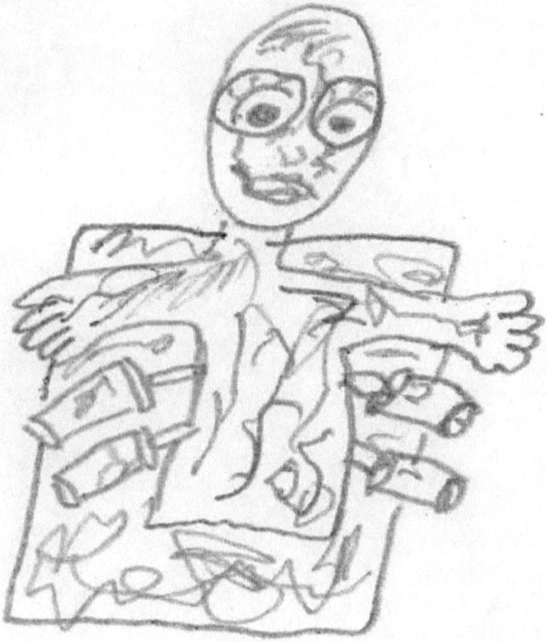

## Cockroach

1. Cut yourself in half at the waist.
2. Amputate your arms and legs at the elbow and knee.
3. Staple your lower arms and legs to your torso.
4. Bash your head against a wall till your neck disappears.
5. Remove spine. Saw it in half and staple the two halves to the top of your head.
6. Cut off hands and sew them to your chin.
7. Now cover yourself in lighter fluid and set yourself alight. Wait till you attain third degree burns then put yourself out.

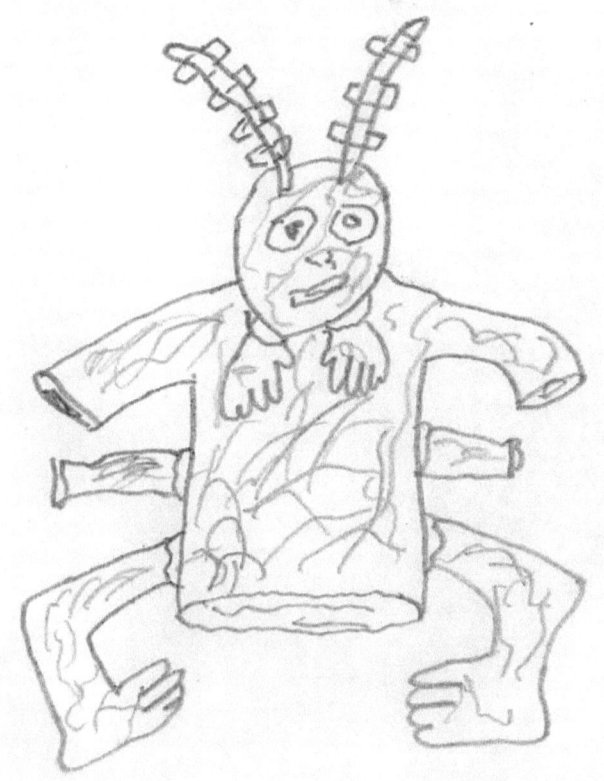

## Cricket

1. Amputate legs.
2. Glue them to the sides of your torso.
3. Cut off your hands and staple them to the space between your arms and reattached legs.
4. Use sand paper to remove all facial features including ears.
5. Cut two thin long strips of skin off your back.
6. Staple these to your forehead.
7. Smack your head against a wall till your neck disappears.

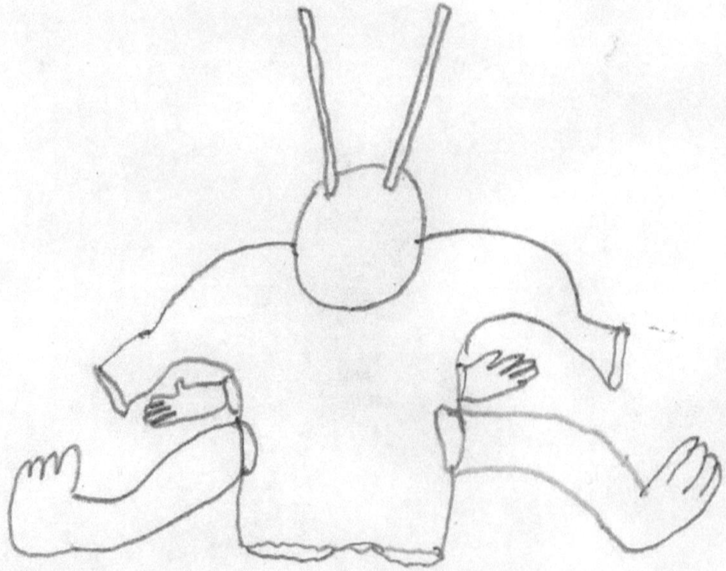

## Fly

1. Cut self in half at the waist.
2. Amputate legs and cut them in half at the knees.
3. Staple the leg segments to your shoulders and the sides of your torso.
4. Use garden shears to remove lower jaw.
5. Use a plunger to collapse your anus in on itself.
6. Snip off your rectum and staple it to your nose.
7. Chisel away at your eye sockets till they are completely broken away.
8. Inject your eye balls with air. Do this about four times.
9. Cut two diamond shapes out of your back skin.
10. Glue these to the sides of your torso.

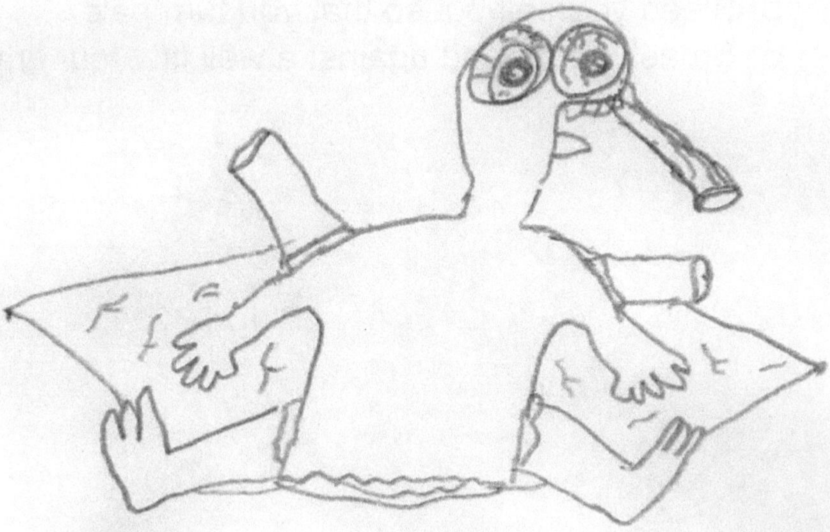

## Gnat

Replicate Mosquito procure. Cut your rectum in half.

## Grub

I looked up pictures of these and gagged a little bit. It's the little arms that get me.

1. Amputate arms and legs.
2. Remove spine.
3. Cut fingers off hands and glue them to your arm stumps.
4. Use sand paper to rub off all your facial features and remove your ears and hair. Go ahead and remove your genitals too. Why not.
5. Bleed yourself out so that you turn pale.
6. Smash your head against a wall fifty four times.

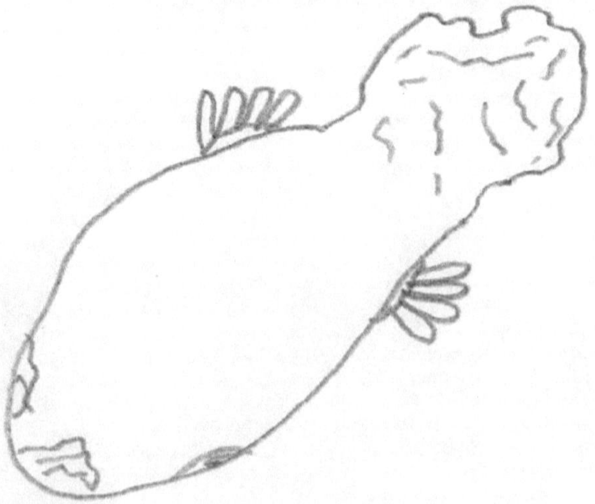

## Grasshopper

(See Cricket. Paint self green.)

## Hornet

See Wasp. Take steroids.

## Ladybug

1. Cut yourself in half at the waist.
2. Amputate arms.
3. Cut three fingers off each hand.
4. Glue these fingers on to the sides of your torso, descending from the top to the bottom. Make sure they are spaced out evenly.
5. Glue your chin to your sternum.
6. Remove all hair from your head and body.
7. Pull out your top teeth and glue to the top of your head in a horizontal line.
8. Use black, white and red paint to create markings.

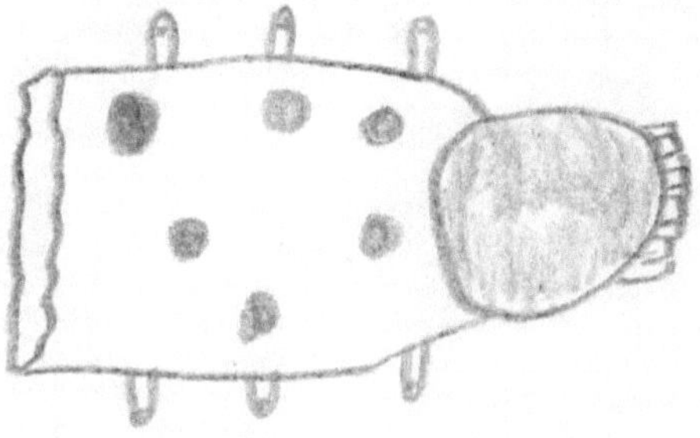

## Leech

1. Remove ribs.
2. Fill a bath tub with hot tar.
3. Position a power saw, sander and hot iron on the floor.
4. Wriggle on the ground into the power sander to amputate your arms and legs.
5. Then wriggle onto the sander to remove all facial features and smooth out your entire body.
6. Cauterize wounds with hot iron.
7. Finally, dive into the bath of hot tar.

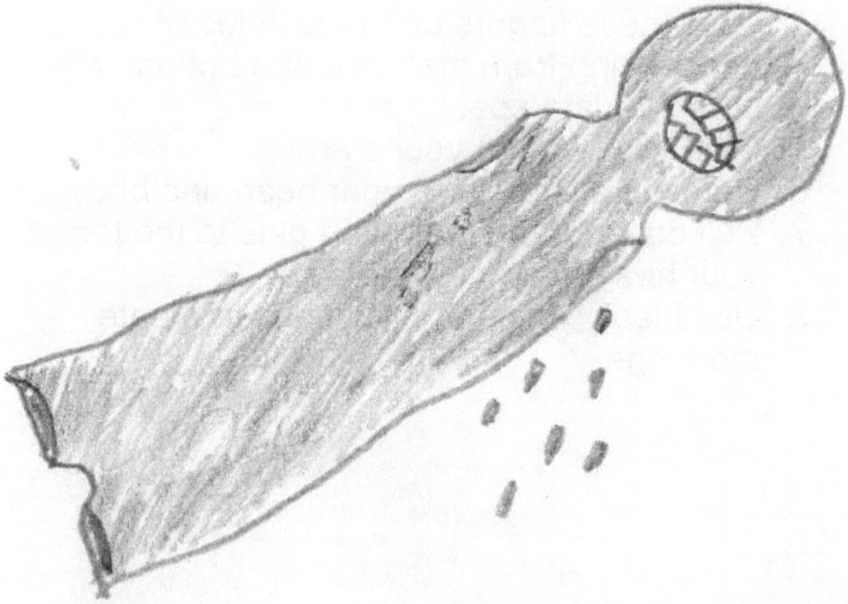

## Maggot

1. Shave all the skin from your body.
2. Remove all the bones from your neck.
3. Push your head down INSIDE your body so that only your head from the upper jaw upwards is sticking out.
4. Use sand paper to remove all facial features.
5. Cut yourself in half at the hips. Disregard bottom half.
6. Use a large knife to score a series of lines up the body.
7. Position a power saw on the floor and use it to cut off both arms.
8. Dive into a bath of Vaseline and emerge, a Maggot.

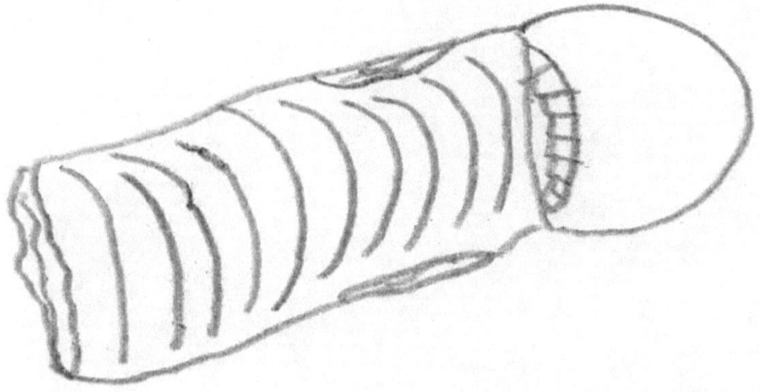

**Author's Note: Forgive my son Steven for making this illustration look so much like a man's spunk trunk. He is so young and unworldly. I for one am proud of my son's magnificent dick drawing. It takes skill to make something like this appear to leap off the page. I love you Steven. Keep em comin'.**

## Mosquito

1. Cut yourself in half at the waist.
2. Use a plunger to collapse your anus in on itself.
3. Snip off rectum and staple it to the bottom of the living half of your body.
4. Amputate arms at the elbow.
5. Glue the severed arms to your shoulders.
6. Use garden shears to remove lower jaw.
7. Pull out tongue. Stretch it out as long as it can go without tearing. Then staple it to your nose.
8. Cleave all the skin and flesh off your limbs.
9. Cut two diamond shapes out of your back skin. Stretch these out as far as they can go without tearing.
10. Glue one end of these to your spine.

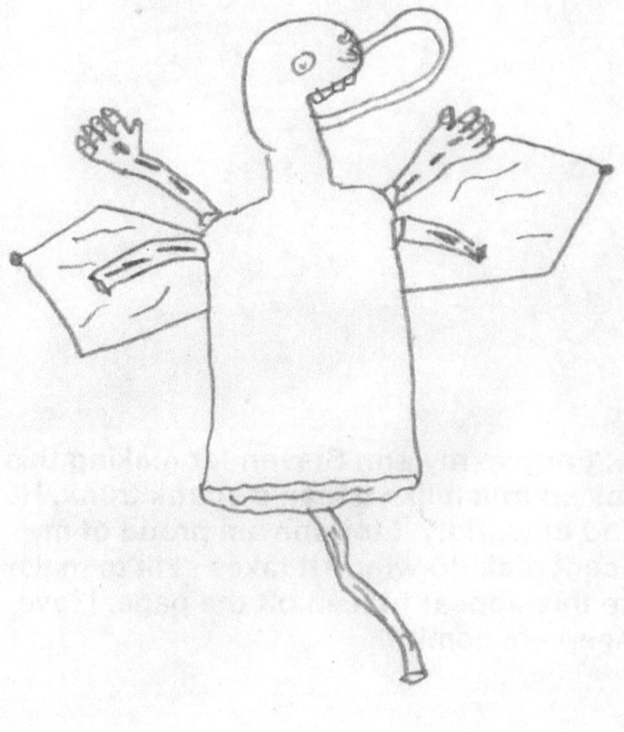

## Moth

(See Butterfly. Choose a less colourful, more faded shade.)

## Scorpion

1. Amputate one foot. Cut the foot off and sharpen the end of the leg into a sharp point.
2. Use a kitchen knife to cut your anus out. Trust me, this will save you a lot of hassle later on.
3. Stuff the top end of the severed leg into your anus.
4. Cut your arms and other leg off at the elbow and knee.
5. Cut off your hands and feet.
6. Copy instructions 3, 4 and 5 of the Lobster procedure in the Sea Invertebrates section.
7. Staple your severed arms to the sides of your torso.
8. Staple your severed leg to the stump where you other leg used to be.

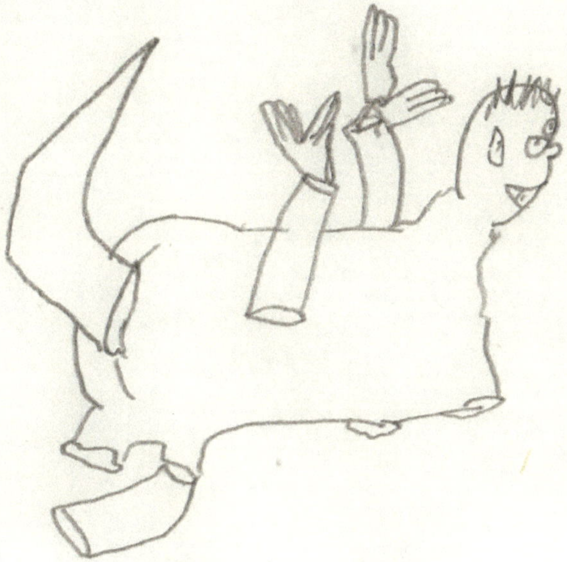

## Slug

1. Sand off all skin till you are left with a layer of sticky exposed flesh
2. Dive into a bath of goose fat or a lubricant of your choosing. This will simulate a slugs natural goo. Keep this bath constantly filled in case you need to reapply.
3. Use a blade to remove eye lids.
4. Gently reach into your sockets and get a grip on your eye balls.
5. Stretch your optic nerve till your eye balls are dangling out of the sockets. (Be extremely careful. Do not pull too hard or you will pull your eyes out completely.)
6. OPTIONAL – Prop up your eyes with two sticks.
7. Saw off all limbs and cauterize stump wounds.

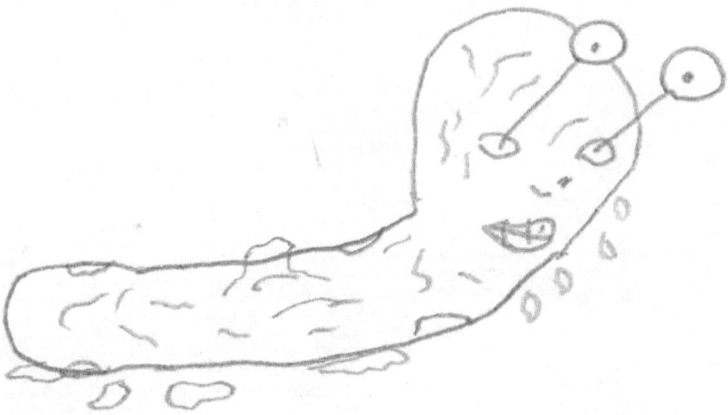

## Snail

(See Slug. Construct giant shell to live in.)

## Spider

*Shudder* as an arachnophobe this was a joyous procedure to think up.

1. Amputate arms and legs at the knee and elbow.
2. Sew your arms to the sides of your torso.
3. Sew your legs to your shoulders.
4. Cut off your feet and staple them to the sides of your mouth.
5. If you want multiple eyes simply glue googly eyes to your face or draw them on with a pen.

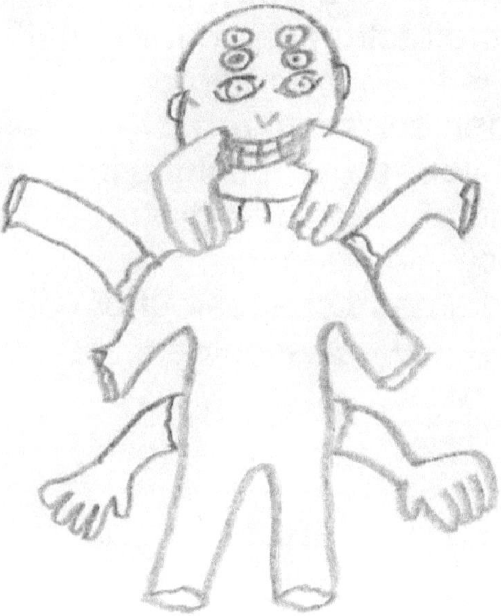

## Tarantula

(See spider. Cover self in hair.)

## Virus

(See Bacteria. Act more malicious.)

## Wasp

1. Amputate legs.
2. Cut the legs in half at the knee.
3. Sew the leg segments to your shoulder and upper sides of your torso.
4. Use a plunger to collapse your anus in on itself. **[I will NEVER get sick of writing that sentence. It's pretty much the basis for writing the whole book.]**
5. Snip off the rectum and cut it in half. Glue the two halves to your forehead.
6. Use garden shears to remove lower jaw.
7. Chisel at your spine, pushing it down your back till the end of your spine protrudes out of your lower back. Sharpen this.
8. Cut two diamond shapes out of your back skin.
9. Glue these to your shoulders.

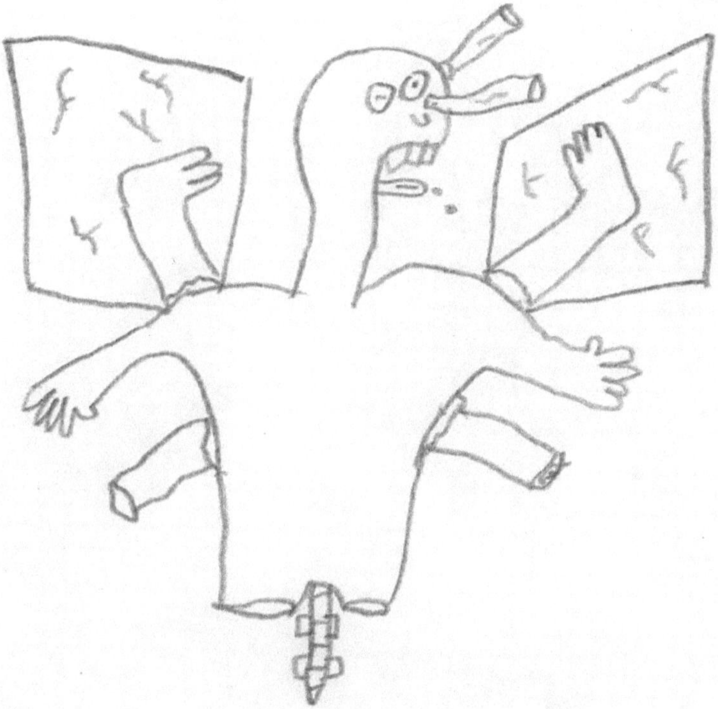

## Worm

1. Shave off all the skin from your body.
2. Remove your ribs and all the bones in your legs.
3. Fuse both legs together.
4. Now the fun part. Get a hot knife and cut a series of horizontal lines all the way up your body. Remember to leave one section in the middle of your body untouched.
5. You need to induce swelling in this middle section. Inject it with dirt and sperm or simply whack it with a club.
6. Sand off all facial features.

7. Amputate both arms.

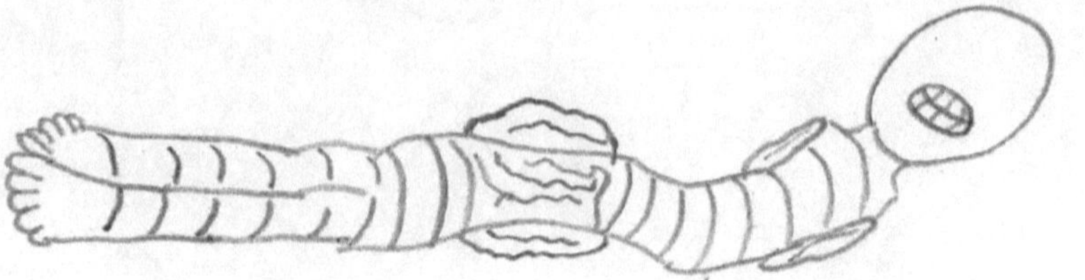

# Section 7: Sea Invertebrates

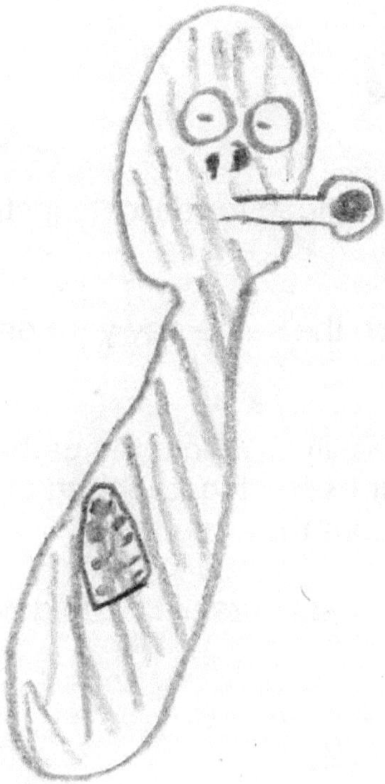

## Anemone

Replicate the Jellyfish procedure.
When you get to instruction 13, dip entire body apart from your brain stem into the shredder. Then swiftly pull your newly shredded body out.
Dive into a barrel of pink dye.

## Barnacle

This one is tricky. You need to replicate instruction 1 of the Coral procedure.

This must be done on the same day your garbage is picked up. Why?

Coz you need to sneakily dive into the garbage truck crusher. Allow it to mash your bones together and once you resemble a barnacle hop out before they see you.

You'll have Transformed yourself on the government's dim! Ha ha ha.

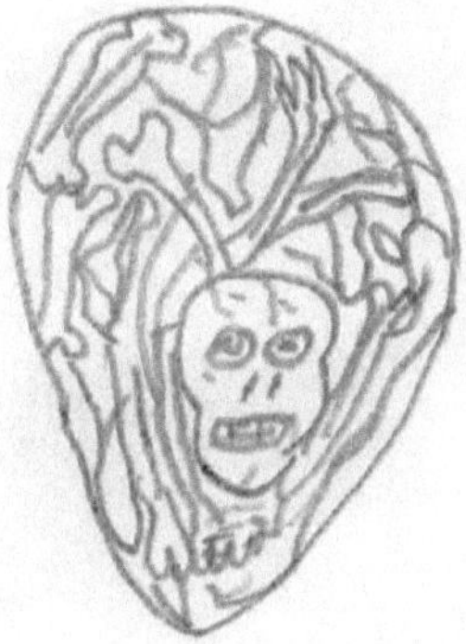

## Coral

1. Use an electrical carving knife and chisel to remove all the skin and flesh from your body.
2. Use a large ballet to obliterate your arms and legs so the bones shatter.
3. Cover the rest of your boney body in super glue.
4. Now roll around on the floor, so that the shattered limb bones stick to you in random places.
5. Dive into a barrel of dye. You can choose your own colour.

<u>Crab</u>

1. Use hot glue to fuse fingers together. Leave the thumb separate.
2. Make an incision down your torso. Use a hammer to break your ribs. Snap them and pull them out of your chest cavity.
3. Remove intestines, spleen and appendix.
4. Push all other organs to the sides to make room.
5. Use a crow bar to wedge your neck bone and snap it clean off.
6. Push down on your head with all your might till it is push down into your torso.

7. Amputate arms at the shoulder.
8. Now cut the arms in half at the elbow. Take the arm half that has your hands attached and sew them back onto your body.
9. Get a hammer and bash in your eye sockets.
10. Pull the eyes out of the sockets making sure the optic nerve is still attached. Pull the eyes out of your torso.
11. Sew your torso back up.
12. Cut off legs at knee.
13. Glue your severed legs and arms to the sides of your torso.

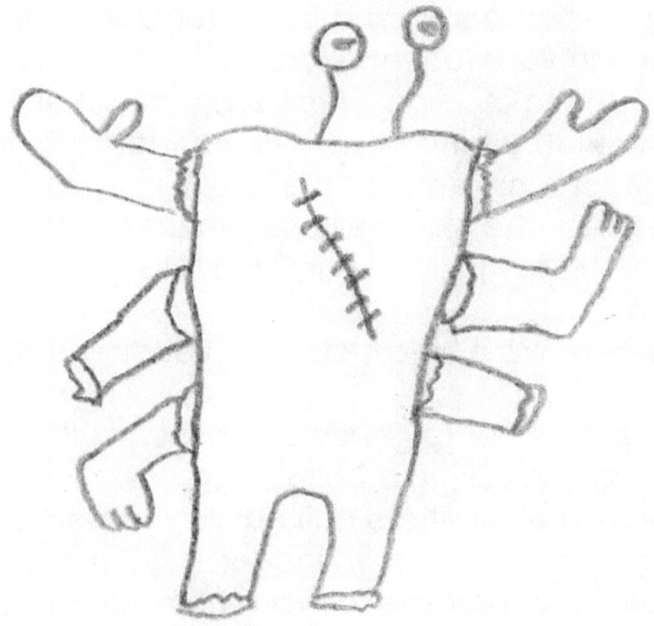

## Cuttlefish

(See Squid. Cut tentacles in half.)

## Jellyfish

This procedure involves systematically removing all the bones in your body.
Before beginning place a shredder and a man sized Breaking Bad style barrel filled with acid on the floor. The acid should be strong enough to give the entire surface of your body third degree burns but not eat through your entire body.

1. Begin by cutting a long incision from the bottom of your foot to the top of your leg.
2. Peel back the skin and begin removing all the bones in your foot and leg.
3. Sew up the incision. Repeat on the other leg.
4. Now cut three incisions into your torso. Connect them so they make a Y shape.
5. Peel back the skin and use a hammer to break all the bones inside your torso. Now remove them.
6. Now remove all the skin from your head and face.
7. Use a hammer to gently crack the skull, as if you were cracking a boiled egg.
8. As you skull shatters pull out any remaining shards that still remain lodged in your head.
9. Repeat this process for your neck, shoulders and spine.
10. When you find yourself completely boneless, sew yourself up.

11. Now slither into the acid barrel. Swim around till the acid completely eats away your surface of your body.
12. Slither out and move towards the shredder.
13. Dip what used to be your legs into the shredder and pull them out when they have become strips of flesh AKA tentacles.

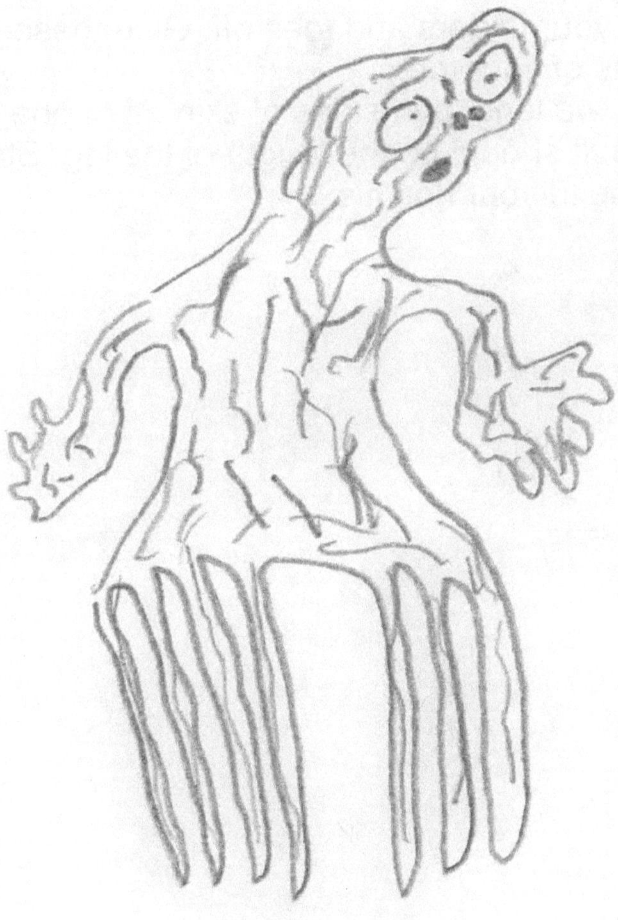

Lobster

1. Cut off arms at the elbow.
2. Cut hands and feet off.
3. Sew them together at the wound so that they make a V shape.
4. Do the same to the feet.
5. Staple the hands to one elbow stump and the feet to the other.
6. Cut body in half at the waist.
7. Cut your fingers and toes off. Glue these to the sides of your torso.
8. Cut two long, thin strips of skin off of one of the legs. It should be the length of the leg. Staple these to your nostrils.

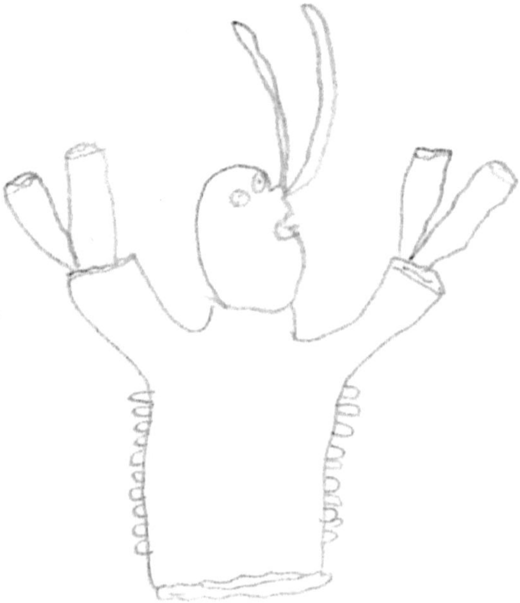

## Plankton

Here you have two options. You can either Transform yourself into a school of tiny plankton or be one massive plankton.

School of Plankton:

1. Position a power saw on the ground.
2. Dive into the saw multiple times until you have divided yourself into about 46 separate small "chunklets" of flesh and bone.
3. Roll around in a mixture of glue and glitter.

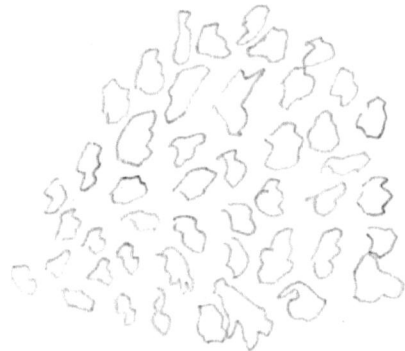

One Massive Plankton:

1. Cut off arms and legs.
2. Use a blowtorch to obliterate your face.
3. Cleave off the skin and flesh from your severed legs.
4. Drill two large holes into the top of your skull.
5. Jam the leg bones into the skull holes.

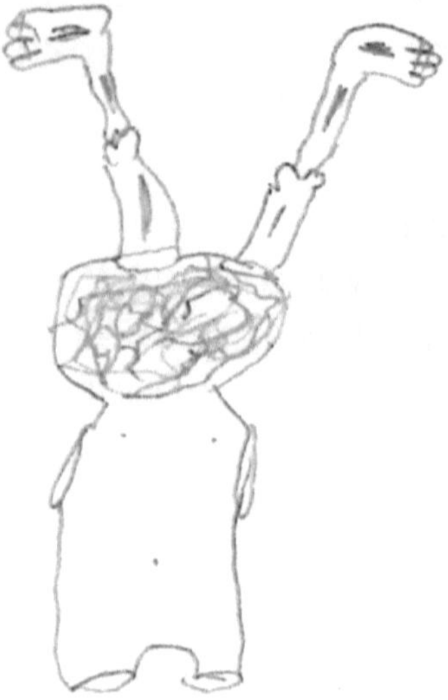

## Prawn

1. Staple legs and feet together.
2. Fall backwards onto a rock. Make sure the middle of your spine lands on the rock.
3. Bend forward and snap your back into a 90 degree angle.
4. Use hot glue to fuse upper arms to stomach.
5. Stick arms in a shredder and pull them out again after about 30 seconds.
6. Pull out teeth with pliers.
7. Use garden shears to remove your lower jaw.
8. Cut two thin and long strips of skin from your torso. They should be the length of your torso.
9. Staple these to your nose.
10. Cut off your fingers and thumbs. Glue them to the sides of your torso.

11. Use a bicycle pump to puff up your eyeballs. Smear black bye on them.

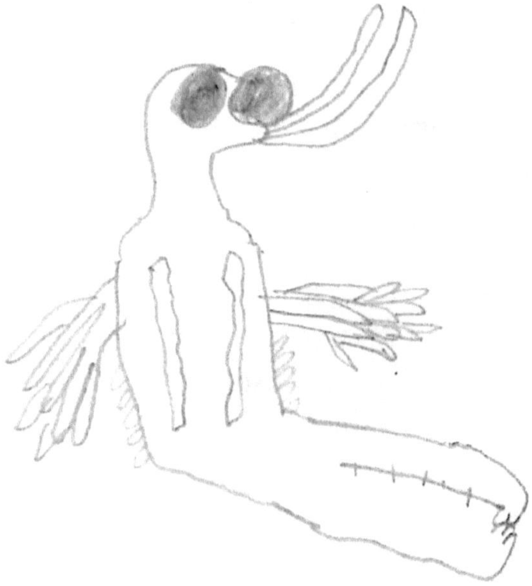

## Shrimp

Replicate Prawn procedure. Use a microwave to compress yourself.

## Sea Cucumber

Replicate Slug procedure.
Cut up spine vertebrae into segments. Stab them all over your body. Use a hammer to make sure they are embedded properly.
Dive into a bath tub of dye. The colour can be your choice.

## Sea Horse

1. Pucker your lips as if you were a cartoon character kissing or Pingu when he goes "Noot Noot". Smear your lips in hot glue and wait for it to set.
2. Stick your lips in a vice and pull your head back as hard as possible so that your lips stretch.
3. Remove all your skin with a good ol' knife.
4. Press a hot iron all over your body till the exposed flesh hardens.
5. Cut off your nose and ears.
6. Amputate both arms and one leg.
7. Remove genitals.

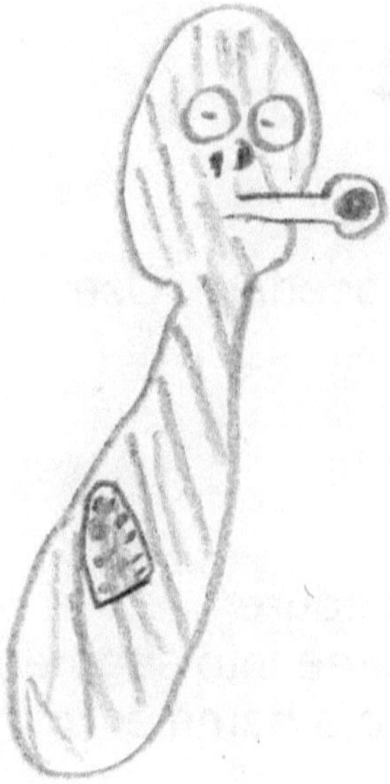

## Sea Sponge

1. Remove all of your skin with a potato peeler.
2. Fill a large pot with water and bring to boil.
3. Dive in and boil self for just under 15 minutes. (Any more and your flesh will get too runny.)
4. Use a fork to fluff up your loose flesh. Then use it to stab holes all over your body.
5. Use a variety of forks and implements in different sizes to stab further holes.
6. Remove all the bones in your neck.
7. Push your head down INSIDE your body so you appear headless.
8. Position a power saw on the floor and use it to amputate all your limbs.
9. And of course do the same thing to your genitals.
10. Bring the pot of boil with a fresh batch of water on high heat. Then turn down.
11. Dive in and let yourself simmer till you flesh has turned from pink to a yellowish white.

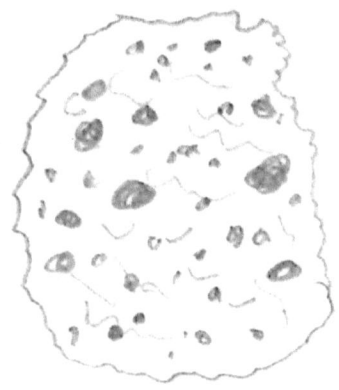

## Sea Urchin

See Hedgehog. Moisten self.

## Starfish

1. Use a power sander to smooth out your entire body, and remove your facial features/genitals.
2. Prepare a bath with boiling hot water.
3. Dive in. Boils should begin to appear all over your body.
4. Get out of the bath and stretch your arms and legs to create a star shape.

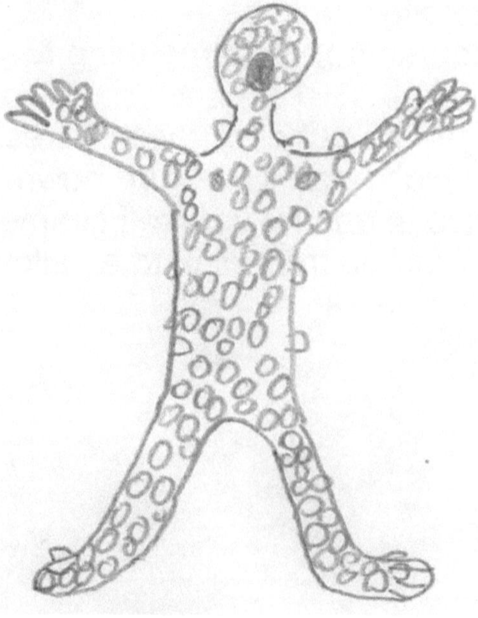

## Conclusion

Well there you have it, a complete guide to Transforming yourself into practically any animal. I do hope this book has been useful to you and that you become the entity you've always wished to be. However, there is one other creature... Something The Man doesn't want you to know exists. But I know they do. I have seen them. I have touched them. I have been interfered with by them. I present to you now a bonus procedure:

## They Who Come From Beyond The Stars

1. Cut off your pinkies.
2. Starve yourself for three months.
3. Remove the top of your skull.
4. Rub a mixture of brown sugar, dirt and semen into your brain. It will begin to swell.
5. Cut off legs at the knees.
6. Cut wrists vertically and bleed out till you appear pale.
7. Apply glow in the dark paint to skin.
8. Remove eyelids.
9. Chip away at your eye sockets with a hammer and chisel. Shape the bone into large ovals.

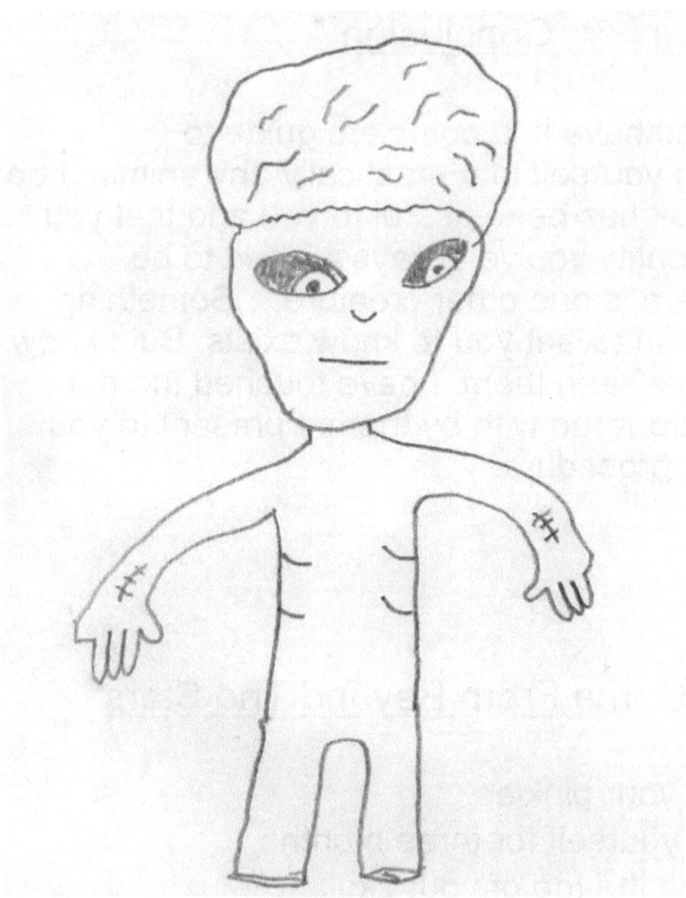

# Coming Soon:

## How to Transform Yourself into Any Extinct Animal

## and

## How to Transform Yourself into Any Object

**Contact Orca Man at: iamorcaman@gmail.com**

**Visit Orca Man's page on the world wide web: www.iamorcaman.blogspot.co.uk/**

**Orca Man is on the Twitter too: @IamOrcaMan**

www.ingramcontent.com/pod-product-compliance
Lightning Source LLC
Chambersburg PA
CBHW021434170526
45164CB00001B/242
*9781507876329*